Tutorial
Therapy

Tutorial Therapy
Teaching Neurotics to Treat Themselves

by

Diana Bovill

Consultant Psychiatrist
Burnley General Hospital

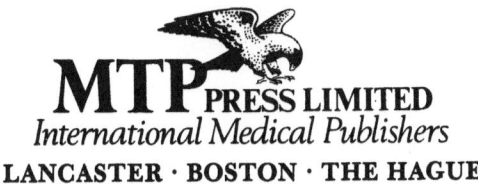
MTP PRESS LIMITED
International Medical Publishers
LANCASTER · BOSTON · THE HAGUE

Published in the UK and Europe by
MTP Press Limited
Falcon House
Lancaster, England

Published in the USA by
MTP Press
A division of Kluwer Boston Inc
190 Old Derby Street
Hingham, MA 02043, USA

British Library Cataloguing in Publication Data

Bovill, Diana
    Tutorial therapy: teaching neurotics to treat
    themselves.
    1. Group psychotherapy
    I. Title
    616.8'5206   RC488

Phototypesetting by Swiftpages Ltd., Liverpool

ISBN-13: 978-94-011-6272-2   e-ISBN-13: 978-94-011-6270-8
DOI: 10.1007/ 978-94-011-6270-8

Contents

Foreword

Dr Bovill is a remarkable person and this book is an eloquent expression of remarkable achievement.

When, some seven years ago, I came to the North West from the relative psychotherapeutic luxury of London, I was amazed to discover a busy whole-time general psychiatrist who claimed that she and her staff were giving a comprehensive service for the treatment of psychoneurosis by psychological means. I did not accept the facts but I believed in the genuineness of the person, Diana Bovill. After careful observation and enquiry, my initial scepticism turned to admiration. I do not know of any psychotherapist who before has provided such skilled therapy for so many people at once.

Another, and in some ways greater, surprise awaited me. Dr Bovill has consistently, dedicatedly, striven to describe clearly, and to evaluate scientifically, her work – an attempt all too rare amongst psychotherapists. Entering psychiatry at a somewhat advanced age, she achieved the rare, and perhaps unique, distinction of being awarded a Doctorate of Medicine at London University for a study in psychotherapy research, approved by the doyen of British psychiatry Sir Aubrey Lewis.

Dr Bovill, unlike many so-called 'experts', does not conceal ignorance under pretentious academic, technical jargon. She has the refreshing gift of expressing herself in direct, down-to-earth and often pungent, language – and is not afraid of being labelled 'naive'. Her approach to therapy was born from deep and often bitter personal experience and she has a once-seen never-forgotten clinical flair. Yet, she has been able to convey her method to many others.

It cannot, now, be said that Dr Bovill's 'tutorial therapy' is idiosyncratic, although it remains to be seen how far it can be practised by her students when she is permanently absent. We must have serious doubts when we remember one of her heroes, that grossly underestimated clinical genius Alfred Adler. Nevertheless, this book, like many of Adler's (written in ordinary language and, hence, ignored officially but quietly purloined by most academics) is a legacy – not only for the 'ordinary' (but always extraordinary) reader who wishes to understand and heal himself; not only for the doctor or non-medical person who is looking for a preliminary guide through the babel of tongues in psychotherapy; but also for specialists who, like myself, do not always share her assumptions and theoretical formulations, and do not practise all her techniques. In the present state of our knowledge, psychotherapy has need of as many approaches as possible – so long as they can be formulated clearly, and might answer to the condition of suffering human beings.

My respect for Dr Bovill's ability, courage and tenderness has, over the years, grown into an abiding friendship – a friendship which is an ongoing dialogue in which we can both say with William Blake 'be my enemy for friendship's sake'. This book does not deal with the subtleties of personal relationships which are so important in everyday life; it grossly neglects two-person situations. Those are only some of my own views about which she and I can half-agree and half-disagree (although, having attended her groups, I suspect that some of the controversy is more verbal than real). But, on some things we always agree – about the importance of providing psychotherapy not only for the privileged few but also for millions of distressed persons in all walks of life, and about the urgent need to combine teaching with balanced methods of assessment.

Dr Bovill's achievements are not confined to psychiatry. An able farmer and gun-dog trainer, she is the only woman to have trained and handled a dog to win the Any Variety Spaniel Championship of Britain – the Blue Ribbon of that field-sport. Often, she compares neurotic human beings to other neurotic animals but, having seen her at work, I have learned much more how dogs, like persons, grow with love. In that, Diana and I agree. She once wrote to me – 'Every patient who recovers is a fresh miracle and the gilt never comes off the gingerbread'.

Robert F Hobson, BA, MD, BChir, FRCPsych, DPM
Consultant Psychotherapist, Manchester Royal Infirmary and University Hospital
of South Manchester.
Honorary Reader in Psychotherapy, University of Manchester.
Director of Training in Psychotherapy, North West Region.

Introduction

This book describes a method of didactic group psychotherapy for the treatment of neurosis. It is generally accepted that the neurotic's education for lifemanship was faulty in some respect. The didactic group psychotherapy method attempts a simple re-education in the areas at fault.

The method owes much to Adler (1929), Pavlov (1926) and Wolpe (1958), and combines psychotherapy with behaviourist methods that patients are advised to apply by themselves and for themselves.

The particular assets of this method are considered to be efficacy combined with economy in therapists', especially psychiatrists', time. The controlled studies reprinted in Appendices (a) and (b) (Bovill, 1972 and 1977) and the review of a year's work in Chapter 12 will enable the reader to judge whether these claims are justified.

As the method is comparatively simple it can be taught to selected and suitable paramedical and lay therapists in a few months, their work as qualified and effective therapists under medical supervision will add to economy in medical time.

This method of group psychotherapy was developed in the provinces where there is the greatest shortage of staff, so time for the active treatment of neurosis by individual psychotherapy or behaviourist methods is available for only a few patients. The great majority of neurotics are managed, rather than treated, with reassurance and palliative medication given by family doctors or junior psychiatrists in busy clinics. Neurotic inpatients may receive some psychotherapy from the ward doctor, but contact is often lost on leaving hospital. Medication and occupational therapy is prescribed, while reassurance and encouragement are given by nursing staff. If these measures fail to discharge the patient in reasonable time then electroconvulsive therapy may be prescribed; the side-effect of this on the memory often breaks up the worry and anxiety pattern just long enough for the patient to be sent home.

Spontaneous recovery, as described by Wallace and Whyte (1959) may also occur; this is often brought about by environmental improvement as a result of medical advice, and the help of the social services. However, relapse is likely if stress arises again.

Such palliative treatments may continue for many years, leaving in their wake unhappiness, disability, absenteeism leading to unemployment, broken marriages and emotionally or physically damaged children. The neuroses of the parents shall be visited on the children unto the third and fourth generations.

In the hope that this state of affairs might be improved by the provision of active treatment I attempted, with some diffidence, to develop a method that would be sufficiently economical in terms of time to enable me not only to treat the neurotics in my care, but to continue their treatment when they left hospital. At the time I was senior registrar in a provincial county hospital where I had the care of the acute admission ward. The more severely affected neurotic patients were admitted to this ward, and many of them had been using the revolving door for years. These early patients provided the material on which I wrote my thesis (Bovill, 1965), and from which developed the paper reprinted in Appendix (a) (Bovill, 1972). Subsequently, the great majority of patients treated by this method have been collected and treated as outpatients.

When I began to treat patients in classes I had no great expectations of the method, having only used it previously on a few patients, treated individually. It was encouraging to find patients responding better in a class situation than they had individually, and learning from each other. Thus another advantage of the method became apparent: patients were treating patients. Years later, in Burnley, when the numbers of patients needing treatment began to grow, the idea developed of training selected volunteers who had completed treatment to act as therapists. Thus a psychotherapeutic 'conveyor belt' evolved.

Soon after I began my class treatment of patients I started to collect data and controls. After 18 months I found time to tabulate the data. I then discovered that the treated patients had averaged 1 day of relapse and readmission to hosptial, whereas the controls had averaged 1 week. I had thus found a criterion for the success of the method. I was astonished and, at first, disbelieved the figures – that so simple a method should prove so effective still surprises me after nearly 20 years of practising it.

I hope that some of my young colleagues, especially those working in the provinces, will find the method of some interest. If the need for active treatment for neurosis under the National Health Service is to be filled, they too will need paramedical and lay therapists working under their supervision. So, in the hope that the book will prove readable to all the above, I have used the minimum of technical terms and included a glossary. Inevitably, some duplication of material has been unavoidable because it may sometimes be relevant to more than one context.

This theory and method of psychotherapy rests largely on beliefs which, though supported by others, are the fruits of my observation and experience of both animals and humans, including myself. In this they are subjective but, with the exception of Pavlovian principles, all theory and practice of psychotherapy *is* somewhat subjective. Thus the proof of the psychotherapeutic pudding is in the 'eating', and as such is inadequate, because puddings depend not only on recipes but also on cooks and the quality of the ingredients.

1

Theory

Pavlov (1926) coined the term 'conditioned reflexes', and trained his dogs to respond to them. In one famous experiment, having trained a dog to differentiate between a circle and an oval, and to anticipate pleasure at the spectacle of one but not the other, he approximated the two figures until the dog was incapable of telling them apart. The dog was then in a situation of insoluble choice and, as a result, became intensely anxious, apathetic, and unable to respond to any learned experimental signals. This state of unusual anxiety and incapacity lasted for a considerable period. Pavlov called this condition 'experimental neurosis'. This experiment and others were repeated with other dogs with the same results, but in fact no dog was found to be 'stable' enough to resist neurotic reaction if sufficient stress were applied.

Pavlov (1926) deduced that conditioned reflexes are essential to the survival of animals, and major disturbances in their patterns cause chronic anxiety.

Liddell (1954), repeating similar experiments on sheep and goats, used very mild electric shocks immediately following the sound of a metronome. The animals learned to lift the leg destined to receive the shock on hearing the metronome. Liddell observed that considerable repetition of this exercise resulted in experimental neurosis without the animals being subjected to any more-complex conditioning. In fact, the neurosis was lifelong, and the following comparisons with their unconditioned fellows were noted: the conditioned animals were easily startled by harmless noises which did not disturb their fellows, their sleeping heartbeats were irregular, and they showed unusual incompetence when the occasion arose to escape from real danger.

Liddell (1954) also worked with very young twin lambs. He found that a lamb subjected to the metronome/electric shock technique in the presence of its quite undisturbed dam suffered no experimental neurosis, while its twin, receiving the same treatment in the absence of its dam, suffered lifelong experimental neurosis. Therefore, one can conclude that one of the main functions of a parent is to teach their young what they need and need not fear, and in so doing conditioned reflexes are established. Thus in these experiments Liddell was exploring the very grass roots of the causes of neurosis.

The experiments briefly described above show that there is an important relationship between conditioned reflexes and neurosis. Wolpe (1958) and others have supported this by the successful use of conditioning in their treatment of neurosis. What can *we* attempt to deduce concerning the nature of this important relationship?

The most striking characteristic of reflexes, conditioned or not, is the speed of response which, in man, is much faster than could be directed by conscious thought. This is obviously a very important survival factor.

Both the wild animal and the domestic animal living close to nature learn many conditioned reflexes in order to survive, developed from a number of sources of information:

1.   Instinct. This first leads the animal to seek the udder and suck. A conditioned reflex for sucking in response to hunger or the dam's call develops rapidly.

2.   Imitation. A lamb sleeps or grazes through the sound of other sheep and lambs calling each other but leaps to its feet and runs with the flock in response to the presence of a barking dog. It did this first in imitation of other sheep, especially its mother, but rapidly established a conditioned reflex.

3.   Experience. A lamb tries to take milk from the wrong udder and is rebuffed by the owner of the udder, so it learns to avoid provoking aggression in animals larger than itself. Ordinarily, non-provocative behaviour is thereafter initiated by conditioned reflex. To give another example: grazing sheep and cattle very rarely tread on the nests of birds such as plovers, though these eggs are usually laid in open pasture. This is probably due to unpleasant experiences of treading on pain-causing objects, such as sharp stones or sticks, establishing a conditioned reflex which prevents the animal treading on anything strange if it can be avoided, even when travelling fast or skipping at play.

4.   Calculation. It is hardly permissible to use the term 'thought' in relation to such simple animals as sheep or cattle. It is present, if at all,

to a very limited degree and is closely related to experience, a process of $2 + 2 = 4$. If the end-result of such 'calculation' is successful, repetition will convert it into conditioned reflex.

The animal, however, is not a robot that acquires a set of conditioned reflexes at an early age and functions on them for the rest of its life. On the contrary, the process of converting new information into conditioned reflexes is a lifelong, ongoing and flexible process, evidently of enormous importance to the survival of the animal; the less thought/calculation it is capable of applying the greater the importance to it of the conditioned reflex system. This can be illustrated by considering an experienced motorcar driver who changes his car only once in several years. At the point of change he suffers considerable inconvenience because the differences in the siting of the controls force him to function on thought as opposed to reflex. Deprived of the capacity for thought he would be incapable of driving the new car.

To the sheep or goat and, to a slightly lesser degree, to the dog or fox, the system of conditioned reflexes is equivalent to a computer program; it is precise, reliable, not rapidly changeable and controls the working of the machine.

I postulate that Pavlov (1926) and Liddell (1954) caused experimental neuroses by 'scrambling' the computer program, thus causing the animal to lose faith in a system on which it had been utterly dependent from birth, both for day-to-day living and swift response to emergency. It could no longer rely on its automatic reactions providing the expected pleasure or pain, safety or danger, hence the chronic anxiety and inappropriate responses.

Man, too, depends on conditioned reflexes – almost everything which he would describe as 'skill' or 'habit' could be described as conditioned reflex. He, too, starts to acquire conditioned reflexes from the moment of birth, but I postulate that it is only these early acquisitions that are capable of causing neurosis. This is because as intellect develops what the child is taught is monitored by *conscious* thought. This ability to reject ideas and attitudes of mind modifies the emotional charge. We see the fully developed pattern in the rebellious teenager.

Take, for example subjecting a 4-year-old child to Pavlov's experiment, giving praise and sweets when a circle is shown but nothing for the oval figure, then gradually approximating the shapes until, over a period of weeks, the child can no longer differentiate between them.

One would anticipate a marked emotional reaction when this point was reached. However, a 10-year-old subjected to the same experiment would simply say, 'I can't tell them apart any more'. Intellect, conscious thought and the capacity to reason would have robbed the situation of its emotional charge; he or she would no longer be emotionally dependent upon an automatically learned response providing a given result.

I am not suggesting that Pavlov's experiment *could* necessarily cause experimental neurosis in a child. There are vast differences between a child in a normal home and an adult dog in an experimental kennel. However, what I am suggesting is that *before the age of reason* a child is able to acquire conditioned reflexes equivalent to those of animals and therefore capable of causing neurosis. It would appear that those conditioned reflexes acquired *before* the age of reason are not subsequently automatically and naturally subjected to reason. Instead they remain part of the mental equipment of the subject, though they may or may not prove harmful to him. In the case of both the young child and the animal it is the profound dependence for security upon the reliability of the conditioned reflex which causes the deep imprinting and intense emotional disturbance when the faith is shaken.

Every young animal is dependent for survival on parent figures, so the parent's approval can provide a powerful lever with which to teach habits of mind (conditioned reflexes), which may not always be in the best interests of the child. Many parents set great store by their child's success.

From treating neurotics we know that a wide variety of faulty habits of mind cause neurotic reactions. In my theory they all have one common denominator – failure (see Adler (1929) and Chapter 13). The success on which the child is trained to depend for approval may be in any sphere of activity – health, intelligence, appearance, manners, parlour tricks, fighting, athletics, religious observance, etc. Praise is given for success and disappointment shown for failure, so the child learns that a certain type of behaviour or achievement will bring the emotional security on which survival depends. Thus an emotionally charged conditioned reflex has been established.

The reader may argue that the individual I have described above could be called a well-brought-up child. I suggest that the difference between the well-brought-up child and the over-brought-up child lies in the parental attitude. If the training is only for the child's good then it is acceptable, but if the training is designed solely to foster parental pride it is wrong, and the stress on the child may well sow the seeds of neurosis. Animals accept their young just as they are and teach them only what they need to know for their own survival. Man alone looks to his children to bring home laurels for himself, and the damage is done because he demands of his child more than the latter can give, causing a fear of probable failure in the future. At some later date the child, now adolescent or adult, fails to succeed in the sphere where he was 'conditioned' to demand success of himself. The methods learned in childhood, which brought success then, now fail to do so. His computer program has not delivered the goods, and because he is functioning on a conditioned reflex, as opposed to conscious thought, he cannot adjust. He loses faith in his ability to cope with life and therefore develops neurotic symptoms.

The conditioned reflex was taught, so the rational approach of the therapist is to undertake re-teaching. By applying intellect to the task of understanding the nature of the problem, giving the matter rational thought and consciously breaking the habit of mind, man can unlearn the faulty habit of mind learned in childhood. He can also apply his courage to the task of tolerating and ignoring his neurotic fears. The combination of the two may never rid him entirely of his problem but, in almost every case, it will bring the problem sufficiently under his control to enable him to live a completely normal life.

The problem of neurosis is, of course, far more complex than I have described it above, which only explains what I believe to be the *basic* cause of neurosis – whether called habits of mind or conditioned reflexes, acquired before conscious thought had developed sufficiently to monitor their acceptance and carrying with them a heavy emotional charge. The faulty habit of mind is almost invariably multiple.

I have so far mentioned only the parent who seeks to make his or her child a symbol of success, but there are parents who regard their children as inevitable failures and bring them up to apologize for their existence. There are also jealous parents who actively teach their children to regard themselves as failures. All, however, are working on the same success/failure axis, as opposed to the natural acceptance shown by the cow to its calf, because the young child's craving for the security of parental approval leads him to seek and find evidence of approval, even though he may have to stretch his imagination to do so. I recall an adopted child aged about 6, whose adoptive parents had produced two of their own children since her adoption in infancy. The child said to me, 'I know Mummy loves me best because she chose me, she couldn't help having the others'. I have no doubt that this child was being kindly and sensibly reared, but her words illustrate my point. I should add that I, personally, attach no blame to parents who rear their children to be neurotic, they do so as a result of their *own* neuroses. The parent who drives his child to seek success does so to pacify his own sense of inferiority.

Unlike other animals, man is able to use his intellect and imagination to modify and thus complicate his neurotic state, hence many more people suffer from neurosis than ever seek treatment. Unfortunately, though they may be unaware of their neuroses this does not prevent the damage they may do. A person may compensate for his unjustified sense of inferiority by taking pride in the wealth of his parents, or the pallor of his skin, or alternatively the snobbery may be inverted. He may escape from his feelings of unworthiness by having grandiose dreams. He may add to his sense of importance, and/or escape from testing situations, by feigning organic illness, while he may or may not be aware of the sham he is perpetrating. He may mentally endow himself with magical properties to compensate for his neurotic weaknessess, and thus develop his superstitions and magic to the point where they occupy his life to the exclusion of almost any other activity. Most dangerous of all, he may attempt to gain control over his fellow men to compensate for his inward feelings of weakness, which leads to strife and, ultimately, to war. This, of course, is not solely a neurotic problem, but is also motivated by the instinct for survival of the race through survival of the fittest (a similar urge drives the stags to fight in the rut).

If one was born in close association with animals; if, from infancy onwards, they were one's constant companions and best friends, one is likely to see oneself as 'brother to the ox', and survival as nature's primary purpose for both man and animals. It is in this field that one strives to solve the problems of psychology, not through the fantasies of Greek mythology however dramatic and intellectually attractive these may appear.

The scientific research available supports my opinion that both Pavlov and Liddell actually *caused* neurosis, a point of considerable importance. Further, they caused neurosis by interfering with an important part of the subject's survival kit. These workers provided solidly based scientific evidence as opposed to merely thoughts, opinions and clinical impressions.

Freud (1933) also contributed vital information when he taught us to listen to our patients. Listen for long enough and you will hear of the particular conditioned reflex established in infancy which is causing the neurotic reaction. This can then be explained and, with luck, a great light will dawn for the patient, and that is the beginning of successful treatment.

Below I describe my theory of neurosis in the simple and practical terms I use when teaching patients. It is often surprising to find how little one needs to teach; sometimes it is as if all that is needed is to prime the pump. A nurse-therapist in training recently said, as have others before, 'I didn't know there was anything wrong with me till I came to work here'. This perhaps illustrates how little may be wrong with the neurotic who seeks treatment. The difference between the seeker of help and 'the man in the street' is often only a matter of where the shoe of life happens to pinch. It is unfortunate that there is still so much shame attached to those who seek treatment. For example, when staying in an hotel I went to have a drink and a word with the barman whom I know slightly. I remarked on the foul weather I had driven through on the motorway. 'I won't use those roads,' he said, 'They terrify me, I feel as if everything is coming in on top of me.' This, apparently, had not always been so; thus, if at the onset of his phobia he had been a lorry driver, he would probably have been referred for treatment, but because as a barman it is unnecessary to overcome that fear, he will probably never seek help.

DEFINITION OF NEUROSIS

Neurosis is a system of apparently irrational fears derived from attitudes of mind learned in childhood, before the child was protected by the capacity to use adult logic – that is, before the age of about 8. This learning may be, and often is, reinforced in later childhood. For example, parental mockery of the young child appears to him, correctly, as a rejection so the much-mocked child learns to fear laughter. If, in his 20s, he finds himself cringing inwardly in the presence of friendly laughter this may seem irrational to him *until the association with his early experience is pointed out*. If that is his only problem (unlikely though this may be), learning awareness of the cause may suffice to cure him.

AETIOLOGY AND PATHOLOGY OF NEUROSIS

Consider three factors: goodwill, inhibition of courage, and self-concept.

Goodwill

Among those who train sheepdogs or gundogs it is an acknowledged fact that a high loading of goodwill is an hereditary characteristic and increases trainability. Goodwill, often called the 'will to please', is so essential a characteristic of temperament in dogs which must, for example, be trained to ignore the instinct to chase, that breeders of these kinds of dogs breed first for this temperament, and then for the physical characteristics which best suit the dog for the work. This particular factor has so influenced the dog-breeding industry that in several cases two strains of the same breed have developed – those bred for work in which temperament is of paramount importance, and those bred for showing in which physical appearance is of paramount importance. Members of the two strains may hardly be recognizable as the same breed. This breeding has developed in spite of the fact that it would be economically advantageous for breeders to produce dogs capable of performing competently in both areas, but the influence of goodwill on trainability is so great that physical appearance must be sacrificed in order to obtain the high standard of training required.

It is reasonable, therefore, to deduce that the child with a high loading of goodwill can also be more easily trained to ignore his natural instincts and urges, for example the urge to stand up for himself and to venture forth into life confidently. This kind of child is sensitive to, perceptive of, and therefore responsive to, the emotional needs of parents and others. This is certainly an asset to its possessor but only if the training for life is good.

However, if the neurotic's life has been sufficiently damaged by the results of his faulty training in lifemanship his associates, including perhaps his doctors and nurses, may be forgiven for failing to notice the underlying goodwill. This, in hysterics for instance, often presents as a facet of attention-seeking – hence the person who does things for others not desired by the recipient, perhaps at considerable cost to himself, and who then weeps or sulks if sufficient gratitude is not shown.

Nevertheless, perception of this goodwill usually enables one to make the differential diagnosis between the neurotic and the psychopath, in whom the congenital loading of goodwill is below average. (Some who are labelled psychopaths, however, will on perceptive examination be found to have average goodwill!)

Inhibition of courage

Unrealistic training runs counter to normal, right-minded instinct and development. It teaches a child to behave in a way which is socially unacceptable in the adult. Thus it is an attempt to produce a 'good' child as opposed to bringing up a child to be a good adult. It daunts and defeats the child, and inhibits the application of courage to the circumstances where it arises because what he feels deeply to be *good* is represented as *bad* by his adult models. He copies adults because, like every young animal, he has a strong natural imitative tendency to help him learn lifemanship from the adults around him.

Take, for example, the newborn deer calf hidden in the heather while his dam is away grazing. He shows no fear of humans and appears to take pleasure in being stroked, but come upon him later with his dam and he will fly from humans because she does, and learn from her actions to do the same for the rest of his life.

Or consider the small boy who repeatedly watches his father batter his mother. His natural instinct is to attack his father in defence of his mother, not perhaps in a spirit of chivalry but because mother represents food, warmth and therefore survival. But terror of his father's size is too great, which is shaming. Confusion is added when, later, his mother asks him to be obedient and polite to the father whom he hates. So he learns that his natural inclinations are unacceptable, and that it is *good* to inhibit courage in the presence of '*force majeur*' and to bully those weaker than himself. But if, in his 20s for example, he batters children, cringes to foremen and runs away when a thug attacks his wife society will condemn him. Or if his loading of goodwill is *too* great to allow him to compensate for his shame and feelings of inferiority by bullying those weaker than himself, he may grow up to evade all conflict, even to the point of being unable to utter an opinion in the presence of his equals or superiors, and for this society will also condemn him. Before he can begin to recover the use of his courage in conflict or potential conflict situations *it must first be explained to him in comprehensible terms how he lost this capacity*. He can then understand that his difficulties are not due to congenital disabilities beyond his control, and this will give him hope and improve his self-concept.

To take another example, the rebellious feelings aroused by a possessive mother's emotional blackmail are smothered in response to the mother's distresses. The motives for shackling the child are represented as care and kindness provided, often in superabundance, in terms of material benefits. Thus the child is surrounded by expensive toys, has only to ask to receive anything he wants; but if he expresses a wish to go and play with the child next door, for instance, mother's tears make a pool on the carpet. The subtleties of this situation are more difficult for a child to cope with than violence or rejection. He may grow up to be a tough, competent soldier or executive, but a weeping wife may bring him to the psychiatrist. This kind of circumstance has inhibited his courage, boldness and self-assertion. The leverage which maternal distress can apply to a young child is hard to overestimate, not only because he is factually dependent on her for his survival so that her preservation in good order is of prime importance to him, but also because his imitative capacity forms a large part of his survival kit and is directed onto her.

In another example, a patient who had been taught to regard his father as invariably right and righteous, even when he was an obvious bully, gave up a good job only because the foreman would sometimes stand watching him. He was not in any way singled out for this treatment, but it caused symptoms of fear that he found inexplicable. Explanation, and a short course of retraining in application of courage to bullies, enabled him to return to work, and he even found himself able to joke with the foreman.

Neurotics are frightened people who need to be taught to use courage in circumstances under which they have not previously done so, though they are often courageous in other situations. The therapist must point this out to them so that they do not think of themselves, nor imagine that the therapist sees them, as cowards in a general sense. The discovery that courage can be used effectively in situations which have hitherto been found intolerable improves the self-concept and aids in rejection of the faulty childhood training.

Self-concept

The inhibited child has failed in courage. Though on one level he accepts this as 'good', on a primitive level he is ashamed and humiliated, and his self-concept suffers accordingly. A child is born without criteria on which to base an opinion of himself, so he adopts the parental opinion. If for any reason this does not appear good neither will his self-concept. Endowed with a poor self-concept he will lack confidence, and may not realize his potential in play or class, so his self-concept deteriorates further; if acquired before the age of reason, it may never be revised. Thus the rejected child, the adored child of whom too much is expected, the overprotected child who is maintained in a state of dependence, the child of parents who are themselves overconcerned to maintain standards or a good image ('keep up with the Joneses'), the child of reserved, unaffectionate or of quarrelsome, terrifying parents, are all liable to grow up with an unjustifiably poor self-concept. They will attempt to compensate for this by seeking approval and success, and are thus overanxious about the impressions they make on other people.

It follows, therefore, that an important curative factor is an improvement in the self-concept. Unfortunately, through prejudice the very fact of seeking psychiatric help is likely to be antitherapeutic in this context. So the therapist must try to minimize the shame felt, in words such as: 'Everyone is more or less neurotic; when we have taught you a bit more about it you will notice it in others whom, up to now, you have thought were more stable than yourself', or: 'You will learn to understand other people so much better that you will be glad to have come for treatment'.

The neurotic equation

The three factors – goodwill, inhibition of courage, and self-concept – dealt with above are all variables, so the matter may be loosely expressed as an equation:

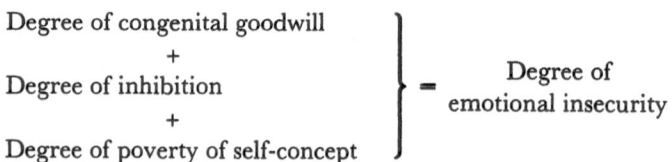

$$\left. \begin{array}{c} \text{Degree of congenital goodwill} \\ + \\ \text{Degree of inhibition} \\ + \\ \text{Degree of poverty of self-concept} \end{array} \right\} = \begin{array}{c} \text{Degree of} \\ \text{emotional insecurity} \end{array}$$

If the degree of goodwill is only slightly above average but the degree of inhibition is gross, the degree of insecurity may be the same as if the degree of goodwill were high and inhibition low. Or again, a child may have a moderate degree of goodwill, be treated kindly but heavily criticized 'for his own good' leading to a high degree of lack of self-concept. Hence some so-called psychopaths, who are low in goodwill though not substandard, and very low in self-concept.

NATURAL HISTORY

Adolescence, the rising sap

In most people the self-concept improves in adolescence. The primitive reproductive drive includes a strong enough urge to fend for oneself to support the young yet to be conceived. This provides a will to succeed in some task be it work, play, or crime. A degree of uplifting admiration from the opposite sex comes to all but the most unlucky. Concurrently, a revised attitude towards the defeats and humiliations of childhood is probably usual, helped by discussion with friends. The degree of improvement, however, varies and may or may not be sufficient to carry one through life. Whether or not it is so must depend partly on the degree and kind of stress to which one is subjected.

Thus the spontaneous improvement in adolescence often causes a gap of 10 or more years between the end of traumatic childhood experiences and the onset of neurotic symptoms. It is no wonder that patients fail to relate the two until they have been helped to do so.

Young patients

Those who are most severely affected retain throughout adolescence the poor self-concept with which their early training endowed them. They have attained no self-realization; their training has played so heavily on their goodwill that they cannot think for themselves and exist only to please others. As most people find this irritating, the more they strive the more they fail. Those who are physically disabled throughout adolescence may fail to benefit from the postpubertal rising of the sap.

Stresses of life

Those in whom the degree of insecurity is gross break down under very ordinary stresses. Others seek help when, as a result of stress, their methods of escape develop to the point of disablement. Some break down when their compensations fail to satisfy, or no longer exist, as in the case of retirement from a job which has represented a status symbol, or the loss of a spouse who has been a prop. The stress which defeats, called the *trigger factor* or *precipitating factor*, is one which reproduces the conditions that led to inhibition in childhood because, faced with such a stress, the patient's courage is inhibited. For example, the man reared by a nagging mother whose wife has taken to nagging will cringe and withdraw, whereas if his workmate nagged him similarly he would laugh or strike out. Cringing and withdrawing lead to inferiority feelings and humiliation, loss of confidence, and thence to escape methods or symptoms of fear, any of which will increase his humiliation thus escalating the condition.

Presenting for treatment

The majority of my patients present for treatment between 25 and 39 years of age. After 25 the courtship stage of marriage is usually over, children are absorbing some of the wife's attention, responsibilities are mounting for both parties, and those in his work are absorbing more of the husband's attention. Fears of unfaithfulness may arise and ageing parents may be making demands. Any of the above may be the trigger factor. The postpubertal tide of confidence is receding in company with the sex drive, these having performed their functions of reproduction and the launching of the young into life.

Another group presents in the 40s; in women the trigger factor then is often the children leaving home, their dependence upon their mother having been her compensation. These patients are sometimes erroneously treated for menopausal depression and the differential diagnosis can present problems. In men, unrealized ambition may be the trigger factor at this age. Only a few patients present at under 25 or over 50 years of age.

THE NEUROSES

Neurotic fear (anxiety neurosis and phobias)

This is neurosis in its simplest form. The symptoms are the physiological signs of fear preparing the organism for fight or flight, though patients often attribute them to disease and rarely know their true causes. The labels attached are often misleading: the *agoraphobic*, for instance, is rarely afraid to walk alone on a moor; his fear in a crowded street is fear of criticism, so he usually feels better alone and in the dark. This is the most common fear, implying a dependence on the good opinion of others which the patient does not expect to enjoy because he has a poor opinion of himself. He is unable to apply courage either in replying to criticism, which is usually anticipated rather than received, or in the normal assertion of personality which carries a risk of rejection but without which there can be no good relationships.

The agoraphobic often feels he has no right to stand idly filling space, but feels more acceptable when usefully employed. Thus a woman may be able to take the child or dog for a walk, but is unable to leave the house alone; or a man may be able to go to work but be unable to go to the pub (though a double whisky taken fast may sedate him sufficiently to tolerate the crowd in the bar, hence some alcoholics).

Claustrophobia is a term used when the fear is of a closed space such as a lift, but again the closed spaces feared are those where there may be other people. I have yet to meet the patient who is afraid to use a small WC. The fear is of having no escape-route from the attacks of other people, so it most commonly arises in larger spaces which it is socially unacceptable to leave, churches and parties for example. Fear of staying alone in a house is often fear of the criticism which may arise if the patient fails to cope adequately with a crisis, a fear liable to occur, for example, when the young wife is left alone at home with her first child.

Fears limited to specific objects such as dogs, mice, spiders or feathers are sometimes the presenting symptoms of an *obsessive compulsive neurosis* (see page 27). Probably these could often be traced to a piece of early training if we could recall everything from birth. Asians, for example, are often frightened of dogs because they have been trained from early childhood to shun them for fear of rabies. To take an animal model: gundog puppies are trained from birth to accept loud, sharp noises. While they suckle the metal feed bowl is deliberately dropped on the concrete floor, the kennel door slammed or a cap-pistol fired. As the dam does not respond with fear neither do the pups. Thus later on they will not be gunshy unless their first experience of gunfire is associated with some other fear.

Fear is an important part of our survival mechanism, so it is certain that no-one can be cured of it. This, of course, is not required in the neurotic because he already knows how to manage fear and is as capable of applying courage as the so-called 'normal person'. Faced with a child trapped in a burning house he is no more likely to be cowardly than any other human being. His difficulties are: (a) that his fear symptoms are mistaken for those of disease, (b) that his fear appears irrational, and (c) that his courage is inhibited in the specific circumstances where fear arises. He later fears the *symptoms* of fear particularly lest they be observed and thus lead to condemnation. This fear of fear causes escalation, hence the panic attack; explanation, therefore, often brings relief while experience of his ability to cope with fear ultimately cures the neurotic of these symptoms.

Neurotic depression

It is socially acceptable to describe oneself as depressed, so patients often use this term to cover any kind of mental discomfort; thus, when taking the history, the question, 'What do *you* mean by depression?' must often be asked. The replies vary so widely as to cover the full spectrum of neurotic symptomatology.

Neurotics are not depressed in the medical sense of endogenous depression. If they respond to antidepressants at all, which many do not, it is usually to the sedatory side-effect of the medication. Neurotics are better described as being unhappy, even miserable, fed-up and discouraged, all of which results from neurotic disablement.

Being frightened is tiring, which is hardly calculated to cheer one up, and having no explanation for one's fears suggests that lunacy is approaching, which is terrifying, so life may not seem worth living. Most of the neurotic's self-destructive actions are demonstrations and/or cries for help rather than suicidal attempts, although genuine suicides do occur.

Escapes and compensations

In its simplest form neurosis presents as an uncomplicated fear, but the child may have learned complex methods of combating fear. Hysteria, the escape into dreams, and obsessionalism, the escape into magic, both occur initially in early childhood in those with hysterical or obsessional personalities. Probably many go through life utilizing these escapes without becoming disabled by them. Escape into drugs, including alcohol, arises in adolescence or later, and only rarely becomes disabling. Hysterics, obsessional neurotics and addicts must first understand that their dreams, rituals or drugs are escape-routes from fear; their situations then approximate closely to those of the anxiety neurotic, and all must learn to cope with their fears.

Hysteria

I do not use this term as one of abuse. In my terminology the hysterical personality is one with a marked tendency to dissociate from reality, substituting fantasy. Hysterical conversion, a dissociative phenomenon, occurs more commonly in those with hysterical personalities than in others.

Congenitally the hysteric has a good imagination and something of a talent for dramatization with its inevitable accompaniment of a liking for the limelight. This has often been denied normal expression through inhibition and a poor self-concept. In childhood the hysteric used these assets to escape from unpleasant reality, thus learning to daydream excessively until his dreams were more important than reality. 'If you can dream and not make dreams your master' – the hysteric is the slave of his. There are both bad and good dreams so he not only compensates for failures by dreaming of success, but also, having read or seen related material through the mass media, he dreams that he will commit murder, is schizophrenic or has cancer. He then suffers severely from fear, but his belief in the reality of his dream will gain him support and limelight which somewhat assuages his suffering. It is difficult, therefore, to persuade him to abandon belief in his dream, so he is more difficult to treat than the patient suffering simple fear symptoms who enjoys no secondary gain.

Obsessive compulsive neurosis

The obsessional personality is organized, orderly, law-abiding, accurate in statements and sometimes gullible, as it is often difficult for him to appreciate emotionally the freedom with which others break laws and make inaccurate statements! He excels in tasks requiring rigid precision and reliability. In childhood these unchildlike characteristics brought him commendation so he cultivated them. Children, like all primitive peoples, believe in magic and are taught to do so through fairy stories and superstitions. The story which tells of someone being commanded to persist in a repetitive task in order to find 'the crock of gold at the end of the rainbow' is the kind of tale which catches the imagination of the obsessional personality because he excels at persistence. So, when under pressure he practises magic as his ancestors have from the dawn of history, and as do millions of 'normal' people who touch wood, throw salt over shoulders, do not walk under ladders and so on. The obsessional *invents* superstitions; he says, for example, 'If I touch every tree on the way to school my sums will be right' or 'If I count every railing on the way home Daddy won't be angry'. In this he is using his natural talents in an attempt to control his environment.

Most children usually reject and forget the magical content of the ritual quite early, but retain the habit of finding comfort from counting, touching and acting repetitively when under pressure. The rituals of the obsessional neurotic are always intended to provide safety, that of himself or some other person. The safety may be of life, limb, health or property, but he only half-believes in the potency of his witchcraft. If he can be persuaded to recover the courage to accept the possibility of disaster, and if it occurs to have faith in his own capacity to cope with it, he will be able to give up practising magic.

I have only come across one obsessional who substituted religious beliefs for the more usual beliefs in magic. She had enjoyed religion in childhood, and the religious concepts linked with the obsessionalism were infantile.

Addictions

The addict is finding 'Dutch courage' and/or 'drowning his sorrows'; most certainly 'The shortest way out of Glasgow is a bottle of whisky'. Whereas the simple-anxiety neurotic is very well-motivated to learn to use courage to recover from his symptoms, the addict knows a faster way of getting rid of his symptoms than any I can teach him. This worsens the prognosis, but in other respects the neurosis, which often led to the addiction, is no different from that of other patients. A congenital tendency towards the misuse of drugs, combined with opportunity, has also been postulated as an aetiological factor.

Minor drug dependency

It is common to see patients who have been on minor tranquillisers, sedatives, hypnotics or antidepressants for many years before they are referred. The difficulty in persuading them to give up taking medication appears to me to be due less to its effects than to the feeling that medication symbolizes someone taking care of them. Again courage, boldness and independence is lacking in this context.

Compensation for poor self-concept

Compensation for feelings of inferiority, because of envy, through professed superiority of sex, race, class, power, money or intelligence probably causes more trouble in the world than any other feature of neurosis or psychopathy. Compensations range from the childish to the criminal through endless permutations. A self-made millionaire, for example, held a party for hundreds on his 70th birthday; he paid the local paper to print a special edition featuring his career on the front page and had a copy dropped at each place at the tables! At the other end of the scale there is Hitler, a psychopath low in congenital good-will, a despised little corporal with an inspired tongue who murdered millions. In advertising, brewers for example use the same principle with slogans like 'He-men drink beer'; some of course then go home to beat up their wives and terrify their children thus perpetuating the myth to themselves that they are, indeed, 'he-men' as a result of drinking beer.

Women often compensate through dependence, seeking pity through self-pity, and destroying their capacity for enjoyment. They feel ill, they weep and plead, they threaten suicide and attempt it, thus bringing upon themselves broken marriages and neurotic children.

2

Discussing Therapy and Method

In my experience the key to the aetiology and treatment of neurosis by psychotherapy is by considering characteristics of courage, rather than sex. Obviously there is an important relationship between courage and sex, especially apparent to those accustomed to handling both entire males and castrates of any species (consider entering a bullock for a bullfight or a capon for a cockfight). Certainly a boy can be trained in such a way as to inhibit him sexually and this can be regarded as either an emotional or partial castration, but before this can be achieved he must first have been inhibited. Thus courage was inhibited before there was any sexual inhibition. Therefore, to aim towards sexual disinhibition is to treat a symptom whilst ignoring the deeper ill. Sexual disinhibition may bring a more assertive attitude towards all aspects of life (just as the restoring of normal sexuality to a bullock would do), with the possible side-effect of generalized disinhibition and recovery of courage. The neurotic man, however, is not necessarily sexually inhibited or, if he is, it may prove impossible to disinhibit him sexually until his courage has been disinhibited; or, if treatment effects the former, he may remain inhibited and unable to assert himself in other aspects of life.

It is interesting to note that all the pioneers of the sexual theories of neurosis were townbred. It is doubtful whether anyone of either sex farmbred and sexually experienced could have evolved these theories for which there are no parallels in the rest of the animal kingdom, and which totally ignore the double sexual function of the female. Her courage, aggressiveness and assertion – that is, disinhibited behaviour

– is more important and likely to be more easily aroused in her function as a mother than as a mate. It is as a mother that 'The female of the species is more deadly than the male'; the male parallel to this role is the fight for the mate and, when courtship and loveplay have satisfied her requirements, her final dominant possession by the male.

If, for the male, treatment can restore normal assertiveness as a result of disinhibition in the context of intercourse, then treatment for the female should be based on disinhibiting her assertiveness in defence of her children, or child substitutes, against her father figures, husband (or husband's substitutes), and not in intercourse where many woman who accept a remarkably passive role derive full satisfaction. If we take, for example, the she-cat or the wild doe rabbit fighting the male in defence of her young whom he wants to kill so she can again become sexually available to him: she is asserting herself courageously and, in so doing, is rejecting his future sexual advances. To this he invariably submits, a complete reversal of the male/female roles as in intercourse.

Human young are unique in that they are commonly reared from infancy under the dominance of their sires. Females of other species reign supreme in the 'nursery' and manage their young without interference from the male (unless he slaughters them in the temporary absence of the female). This position remains until the male young reach puberty, when they present as his sexual rivals. The males of many species help to feed and/or protect the young, but we have no reason to suppose that in so doing they dominate either the female or her young. In contrast, the human male commonly dominates his young either directly or indirectly through his dominance of the female; from her the young of both sexes learn, if only by imitation, that the adult male is dominant in the family and that conflict with him can be dangerous. Although in adolescence they often break away from paternal domination, they are likely to perpetuate this pattern in marriage. Hence we find comparatively commonly the apparently inadequate, submissive woman who is emotionally unable to stand up either to her husband or her boss even in justifiable defence of her children or her interests. We can only speculate on the origins of this pattern in the dawn of human existence, but the perpetuating factor is the human female's basic incompetence as a physical fighter which far outweighs changes in the law and state aid towards equality. If judo and karate were compulsory subjects for schoolgirls, battered wives or children, and maternally spoilt sons would be rarer because the human female would then be on equal footing as a fighting unit with her sisters in other species and thus would gain in her self-concept. Females of any species do not often fight, but if necessary they can do so effectively, so their courage is rarely inhibited in relation to their own species.

In treating the inhibition of courage and self-assertion the therapist is striking at the root of the problem. Moreover, simple explanation of aetiology and the aims of treatment can be offered at the initial interview, and are acceptable to the patient without straining his credulity or intelligence. This would not be so in the case of an analyst attempting to explain the mysteries of anal and oral sexuality, the id, the ego and the superego to a patient with an IQ of say 80–90.

It is my belief that the patient will suffer no harm as a result of being told by the therapist what is wrong with him, and why he behaves as he does and suffers the symptoms which trouble him. Perhaps the origin of the idea that this is harmful results from the *patient's* belief that his symptoms are due to his sins, *or at least to that in himself which he regards as sinful*; he will, therefore, reject and resist, thus causing delay in treatment, so one view is that the therapist should remain enigmatic while the patient gropes. I have found it simple and effective to preface explanations by saying that of course none of it is the patient's fault, anyone would have been/done the same under the same circumstances. This requires frequent reiteration during treatment, especially individual treatment; in group treatment the other patients talking openly of their fears, their attention-seeking and compulsions reduce the shame felt by the newcomer.

As a result of explaining so much to patients I have been accused of over-direction leading to interference with the subject's freedom. I am, of course, careful to start an explanation by, 'I think, but I may be wrong . . .' or, 'Do you think . . .?' And neither my patients' opinions nor my experience support the accusation. I am often the first person against whom the assertion of freedom is addressed and, of course, welcome it verbally.

Moreover, patients absorb no information for which they are not ready; it is common experience to offer the same explanation to a patient on, perhaps, a dozen occasions, and on the last elicit the response, 'That is what I needed to know, why didn't you tell me sooner?' Neither do patients accept explanations without thought; it is also common for a patient to say, 'Last time you said . . . but you were wrong, it's not like that it's like this . . .'. This is progress, as he is thinking for himself and is praised for it, but it was my erroneous explanation, or his misunderstanding of what I said, that made him think.

Other criticisms levelled at the method, usually by those who have not seen it in action, have been that (a) it is a waste of time because neurotics will attend just because it is there and not with any hope or likelihood of improvement; and (b) it will encourage dependence. The answer to such objections must lie in research such as the controlled study (see Appendices (a) and (b)). In fact, regarding (a) above, many patients make great efforts and sacrifices to attend for treatment, and those who suffer panic attacks on public transport but have no other way of travelling show great courage.

To answer (b), there is a grain of validity in the theory that the method might encourage dependence in that a very few patients get hooked on group attendance. But the method lays great emphasis on independence, sometimes succeeding to the point of arousing relative complaint, and it is more common for patients to seek discharge too soon than to need encouragement to be discharged.

A different kind of criticism is sometimes expressed by the experienced psychotherapist who attends a tutorial as an observer and says, 'I don't know how you stand the strain!' Admittedly, 2 hours spent teaching eight to ten patients, each presenting a different aspect of the problem and with a different IQ, background and attitude of mind, is tiring. I rarely undertake a session from 7.00–9.00 pm without spending an hour on my bed in preparation. The principles, however, are so simple that I would hardly describe the method as difficult for the therapist, unless he or she felt that he/she had to know all the answers and could not afford to make mistakes. The intention of the method is to provide psychotherapy for the masses; it is designed as a conveyor belt, mass-production job, and therapy is likely to be better than the lack of treatment which is the psychotherapeutic alternative for the great majority. So, though the concentration needed is tiring, the therapist is under no great strain.

A tutorial might be described as a psychotherapeutic self-service store, where ideas and suggestions on a number of problems and subjects are verbalized in the course of the meeting. It is an observed fact that patients pick up only what they want and for which they are ready, rejecting information for which they are not yet ready. Knowing this, the therapist can talk freely without fear of imposing suggestions which might be harmful, so long as he avoids criticism of a patient and, on the rare occasions when this is needed, puts down firmly the patient who attempts criticism of a fellow-patient. I have found it positively beneficial to say to a patient, 'I don't know, I haven't worked that one out yet, let us see if we can work it out together'. And I make a practice of saying, 'I'm not Solomon, I have no crystal ball, I can only make suggestions born of some knowledge and experience of how people behave and react, but you must decide whether these suggestions fit *your* case. Even if they don't they may help you to find out for yourself what does fit.'

An important feature of this method is the emphasis on the therapist's explanation and description, as opposed to the psychoanalytical principal of non-participation, or participation limited to interpretation of material arising in undirected patient conversation. No therapist can avoid conveying opinions to the patient, but those he does convey, being coloured by patient expectation, may not be those he actually holds. His very failure to speak is liable to be interpreted as rejection. Failure to give and explain a diagnosis is likely to be taken by the neurotic patient as the doctor's ignorance, superiority or arrogance, or the doctor withholding a truth too awful to be borne. So, knowing that even silence will convey inaccurate information, I use direct verbal methods tailored to combat probable patient expectations. I do not always succeed.

Like all psychiatrists I see a fair number of my colleagues' failures, as they do mine. As a result of explaining, describing and 'capping' it is not uncommon, towards the end of the first interview, to hear a patient say, 'You are the first doctor who seems to understand!' What the patient actually means is that I am the first to have expressed understanding in simple terms.

Initially, I used the group method to save time. I often saw, say, three patients individually in a morning and said the same thing to all of them. Experience has since taught me that group methods have far more in their favour than that. Most patients come believing that their symptoms are uniquely shameful and verging on lunacy; so the discovery of a number of quite ordinary people complaining of the same symptoms brings great relief. Patients nearing discharge are encouraging to newcomers. Patients pick up points concerning other patients that I have missed, and the discourse of one patient verbalizes the problem of another who then says in tones of discovery, 'But that is just like me!'. The group can be used to support the therapist's contention that the patient is right, but if the therapist leans too hard on a patient the group will come to the patient's defence. Dependence tends to be on the group rather than on the therapist, which is a step nearer to normality because we all depend on our neighbours; man is a herd animal. The patients are nearly always supportive and rarely aggressive to each other. In this they take their tone initially from the therapist. They learn that the whole world is not against them, and then realize that if the group accepts them so may others, which stimulates them to attempt a normal social life to ultimately replace the group.

In my opinion the method is tough; 'You have to put up with it' is the phrase probably most often on the therapist's lips. Patients are always advised to go out and look for their fear symptoms and reproved if they fail to do so. But failure to attend, or to pay attention (in other words wasting NHS resources), are the only patterns of behaviour for which the therapist infers blame. Medical and paramedical observers have also considered the method to be tough, but the acceptance rate amongst neurotics with no added complications is 90 per cent of those who have attended at least once. In my opinion, most people underestimate neurotics who are, in fact, likely to be tougher in the face of suffering than 'normal' subjects because they have suffered and are suffering mental tortures and the scorn of their fellows. 'Pull yourself together' is the advice most often offered: but how?

To take a wartime analogy: I believe that 60 sorties was the maximum asked, and 90 sorties the maximum allowed, for bomber air crews in the second world war. That is, 90 periods of *intense fear* endured with the compensation, albeit small, of knowing that one was earning the respect of one's fellows and that there was a limitation to the agony. Any patient who has had an anxiety neurosis for a year is likely to have suffered many more hours of fear than that, while despising himself for his apparently irrational fear, and having no reason to believe that there will be an end to his suffering. During this period he has usually coped with life at least to some extent. It is doubtful whether hysterics and obsessionals suffer any less. Moreover, it is often noted that neurotics endure physical suffering and danger with great fortitude. Is this perhaps because it represents a tithe of the suffering to which they are accustomed? Even those who feel justified in scorning and condemning neurotics for being neurotic have to admit that most of them are tough.

It is on this toughness that tutorial therapy relies, and most neurotics like and accept it because the assumption that they are capable of being tough goes some way towards restoring their self-respect. They say, 'I will do anything, but anything, to get over this', and I say, 'Good, because I am offering no primrose path, but blood, sweat and tears'.

Take, for example, a lady nearing 60, by no means an Amazonian type, abandoned by her husband and living alone, who told me she had been unable to go out of doors by herself in daylight for some years. But, if, in the night, she heard suspicious noises she invariably went outside to see what was going on and to protect her property. Certainly one could not regard her as a coward, but could one even justifiably describe her as a 'nervous type'?

Some do not agree when I assert that adult man does not *need* love – he likes it when it comes his way, but this is no indication that he needs it. With the exception of pets that we train to seek love, no adult animal seeks or needs love as opposed to sexual satisfaction, certainly not those living in or near the natural state. Are we to assume that, in this, man is unique in the animal kingdom? Is man and only man incapable of out-growing the infantile need to be loved?

3

Aims, Methods and Therapists

AIMS

The aims of tutorial therapy are to explain the neurotic disability in terms of faulty training for life. This reduces shame, fear, bewilderment and a sense of inferiority in the face of an incomprehensible syndrome. Other aims are as follows:

1. To teach the patient to see those in authority, especially the therapist, as useful servants.
2. To recognize that his goodwill renders him vulnerable to the depredations of others, against which he should guard.
3. To apply courage in circumstances where it is inhibited.
4. To improve his self-concept. To understand himself better, including his escapes and compensations, and thus to understand others better.
5. To attain and enjoy emotional independence.
6. To regard life as an adventure, thus accepting that security, emotional or material, is a mirage.
7. To assert himself appropriately or to refrain from doing so through pity or expediency, but not through fear.
8. To accept death as inevitable, and cross that bridge when he comes to it.
9. To be prepared always to accept the worst that may happen in any given set of circumstances, even if this includes major tragedy; and to do so not lightly but sincerely, finding that this may do much to avert disaster.

10.   To learn to cultivate the habit of happiness.

11.   To appreciate that aggression is not a dirty word but an important tool of life, without which no-one so much as scrubbed a floor properly.

12.   To accept that life is often a matter of making the best of a bad job and liking it.

13.   To abandon escapes and compensations in favour of facing life as it is, and himself as he is.

14.   To learn to accept and like oneself.

Inevitably we often fall short of these aims, perhaps through our own areas of ignorance. No therapist can teach what he has not learned to apply to his own life.

METHODS

This method of psychotherapy has two main themes, explanation and retraining. Explanation owes much to Adlerian and Pavlovian principles. Retraining depends on self-application of behaviourist principles as described by Wolpe (1958).

Explanation

Initially, the therapist must explain the origins of neurosis in the childhood training. A child is dependent for his survival on those training him so his need for their approval is very great. Whether the training is right or wrong, he is highly susceptible to it. Further, all young animals are endowed with imitative tendencies to help them learn lifemanship from adults. The young child's experience of life and capacity for logical thought are limited, which increases his vulnerability to the ideas and opinions of others. The emotional leverage applied by other people is greater if the child is sensitive to the emotional needs of others, as is so if he has a high loading of goodwill.

When these generalities have been understood, explanation must be tailored to relate the individual's habits of mind acquired in childhood to the current apparently irrational fears. When they have learnt this patients often become skilled in working out for themselves the origins of their neurotic reactions.

The patient is taught to remember what has been passing through his mind immediately before the neurotic reaction occurs, and then try to link this with childhood experience. For example: a man who had a panic attack when looking in the window of a bicycle shop recalled that, in childhood, his bicycle had been a frequent source of conflict with his father.

The therapist describes and explains the physiological symptoms of fear and their rationale for preparing for fight or flight. This reduces the fear of fear by helping the patient believe that his symptoms are neither those of physical disease nor incipient lunacy.

An explanation of hysterical manifestations is given to those who present with these. It is reasonable for a person who feels himself unable to cope with life without the emotional support of others, to seek attention constantly, maybe by making emotional scenes, by believing himself physically ill when he is not, or, in extreme cases, by hysterical conversions. The therapist points out that the patient has not invented or imagined his feelings or symptoms; to him they *are* real. But it is also explained that they are precipitated by fear and are usually, in fact, the symptoms of fear or of tension caused by fear.

Obsessional rituals are generally readily accepted as being inspired by fear, because many of them obviously are so. Persuading the patient to break the habit by being prepared to live dangerously can, however, prove very difficult, but not usually impossible.

Alcoholism is also easily explained, but as mentioned in Chapter 1 above, unfortunately the alcoholic has learned a quicker way of getting rid of fear than any I can teach him. Moreover, the pub is often the only social circle he knows, so his habits are difficult to break.

If the onset of symptoms was sudden the precipitating factor is usually obvious, known to the patient and, as Adler (1929) maintains, it is failure, or fear of failure due to taking on added responsibility. What presents to an individual as failure naturally varies with childhood training. If the onset is insidious, this may be due to a series of minor failures in various fields of activity gradually eroding confidence. The explanation here is that the spontaneous improvement in drive and self-image during adolescence accounts for the gap of years between childhood experiences and the onset of symptoms.

Desensitization

Using behaviourist principles we teach the patient to desensitize himself, actively as in the agoraphobic's daily walk, and intellectually in the conscious contradiction of inferiority feelings whenever they arise.

The patient should *seek* fear in order to learn to cope with it but, at first, endure it for very short periods, thus avoiding reinforcement of the habit of fear in the given circumstances. (Not all agree with this latter concept; see Marks, 1981). He should take a pride in his growing capacity to use his courage. Care in giving advice is sometimes required to find methods which are not dangerous, as in the case of someone with a traffic phobia. Inventiveness may be needed as, for example, a patient who could not handle knives for fear of stabbing her child was advised to dress a cushion in the child's clothing and try to stab that. This way she learned that she was unable to perform the action of stabbing her child.

Desensitization of feelings of inferiority includes learning to notice small things that are daily performed correctly and are taken for granted, for example, shaving. The therapist suggests that the patient review the happenings of each day, giving credit where due and maintaining a sense of proportion over the debit items. Advice is also given to look at others with just criticism to see that they too have faults.

Commendation

A therapist must never miss a chance to say 'Well done' – when courage has been shown, when homework has begun to improve the self-image, when thought has been applied to a problem, and when a fresh aspect of the neurosis has been discovered.

Self-abreaction

The patient is advised to recall traumatic childhood experiences and picture them in his mind as if watching a filmstrip. While doing so (in private) he allows his emotions free rein because only thus will the 'filmstrip' approximate to the reality of the trauma recalled. When calm he should assess the content of the 'filmstrip' using logical thought to assess and judge the behaviour of the 'actors'. He should ask himself whether those in authority acted sensibly and/or kindly under the circumstances.

The sting can thus be drawn out of memories which until then have been shaming. This improves the self-image.

Rebellion

Patients who are still allowing themselves to be bullied or taken advantage of are advised to rebel against this. They are, of course, very afraid to do so because, having a poor opinion of themselves they strive to gain the good opinion of others without appreciating that this only inspires scorn. As it is very difficult for them to rebel until they have lost their tempers, which is likely to lead to a family row, they are taught how to rebel passively.

Rebellion, however, may occur in a spontaneous burst of temper which leaves the patient ashamed and frightened. The patient is then reassured that he has nothing to be ashamed of, and that his outburst was part of the normal process of recovering the capacity to assert himself. Those who fear that they may be homicidal in their temper are reassured that many people have passed through this stage in treatment without any of them doing physical damage to another.

Having mustered the courage to rebel and discovered that, given time, they thus gain the respect of others, their self-image is improved, and they no longer present themselves as doormats.

Reassurance

Reassurance is never given for anxieties, including hypochondriasis; doing so is like trying to fill a bucket with a hole in the bottom. Moreover, such reassurance is a dangerously addictive drug, leading to dependence on the therapist which though perhaps flattering is anti-therapeutic. If a patient says, 'When I get this pain I think I am dying', I reply, 'If you are dying you will have to put up with it like anyone else'.

Conversely, reassurance is given freely, though robustly, as recovery from neurosis progresses (though perhaps 'recovery' is the wrong word). Patients are assured that many have been treated by this method before and have benefited so far as to be able to live entirely normally. Therapists do not promise the total disappearance of symptoms; on the contrary a residue of symptoms is probable for a long time, perhaps for life. However, if patients strive to learn what is taught and to follow instructions, they will cope with their symptoms, and when they are confident of doing this they will no longer need to run away from symptom-provoking situations, and their symptoms will gradually fade.

I point out that it does not matter to the sufferer whether the symptoms disappear, or whether the subject becomes so tolerant of them that he can ignore them. From my own experience, I have said to patients: 'I remember the first time I had a panic attack and didn't care. I had been having them for some time but, recently, had been treating myself by the methods I advise you to use. I was on a bus when I had this panic attack. I sat there happy. I have never been more pleased with myself. This method of treatment I'd thought out was working! I could cope with this panic attack, I could just let it happen. Fear of panic was never again going to stop me doing anything I wanted to do. The enemy was conquered, I could cope with fear.'

For a therapist to admit to previous personal neurotic difficulties is undoubtedly beneficial to patients. 'What you!' they say with astonishment, 'I would never have believed it.' I reply, 'Yes, and if I could get over it so can you'.

Patients need the reassurance of human weakness in the therapist. Without this, the therapist's image, especially if he is a doctor, is too self-assured to be therapeutic. The therapist appears to them as the personification of successful human authority, while the very fact that they are in need of psychiatric treatment reduces them in their own eyes to the status of a worm. The gulf is too wide to bridge. So unless the therapist is prepared to admit to experiencing the apparently irrational fear patients feel, the latter will be disinclined to take the therapist's advice.

Phobias of mice, spiders, thunder, etc. are very common. So irrational fear is a common human experience, probably so common as to be universal to some degree and in some context. Thus it should not be impossible for any therapist possessed of honesty and self-knowledge to admit to it. Of course, he would do well to first treat himself before treating patients, because only then will he know what he is asking of them.

Problem-solving

Patients often pose problems concerning their own relationships. The therapist's advice involves a new way of looking at both problem and relationship. As a result patients learn to solve problems for themselves. At first they describe their solutions and ask for confirmation. Later they only mention them to illustrate a point to another patient.

It is usual for a problem in relationships to spring from the patient's belief that he is always in the wrong in any situation involving disagreement. At a tutorial the details of such a situation are discussed and the opinions of other members of the class called for. These opinions are sympathetic to the patient, though perhaps he could have handled the matter more wisely had he been less frightened of condemnation. This is explained but not criticized.

The teaching of rebellion, both passive and verbally active, together with the practice of self-abreaction and improvement in the self-image, all play a part in overcoming the patient's inappropriate reactions when confronted with aggression. Thus he learns to stand up for himself which improves both his self-respect and his relationships.

Authority

Most patients fear authority, and therefore the therapist. So the latter should only exert authority in relation to the patient's contractual obligations and explain this in terms of the need to conserve NHS resources. He should point out that in other respects he is the patient's servant, paid to give treatment.

Under democratic conditions authority is always the subject servant and though, hopefully, may often be respected deserves no veneration. A director runs a business, and in so doing serves his employees. The police control traffic and crime, so to the ordinary citizen they are more useful than repressive. Authority, then, is to be used, not feared.

Criticism

Criticism most often springs from a sense of inferiority. The old criticize the young because they are jealous of youth. Parents criticize children because they want them to be better than other people's children. The boss tears a strip off a husband, who then does the same to his wife.

Man is a herd animal so his normal behaviour is friendly. When criticized he should first seek the cause in the criticizer's mind, assuming, of course, that the criticism was not actively provoked.

Dreams

Those with recurring dreams or nightmares can gain in self-understanding if helped to interpret them. First, it is important for the therapist to discover what the symbols in the dream mean to the individual patient – a cat, for example, may be either a marauder, a filthy beast, a male sex symbol or a loved pet. If and when the interpretation satisfies the patient he can be freed from a recurring nightmare. I advise him to recapitulate the interpretation immediately before going to sleep, reminding himself of the great differences between his circumstances at the time of the initial nightmare and his current situation. If this information is fed into his mind just before sleeping it will return to abort the nightmare by association of ideas.

Take, for example, a young woman who described a frequently recurring nightmare in which she was in a cage with vertical bars; the top was open but she could not get over the sides. She felt herself to be in great danger and would wake in panic convinced that she had only just escaped death. A glance at her record told me that the cage was a cot in the children's ward where she had been treated for a tuberculous hipjoint for about 2 years from the age of 18 months. Abandoned amongst strangers who applied painful treatment by force, as they had to, she of course believed that she was going to be killed. Any young animal would have held the same belief, and its own vain struggles would have reinforced the belief by increasing the force needed. The nightmare did not recur after interpretation and explanation.

Thinking

Delays in recovery are caused by a patient's inability to think for himself resulting from an over-authoritarian training for life. The opinions he utters are those of others and designed to please his hearers. As far back as he can remember he has never thought for himself, so he is unaware of his disability, and trying to explain it is like explaining colour to those born blind, but the atmosphere of the class and the tone of the discussions tend to lead the patient towards independence. The question and answer method is in constant use and, when a patient replies, 'I don't know', the therapist often says, 'Naturally you don't know: but what do you *think*?' If the answer comes back in terms of, 'My husband/mother/wife/father says . . .', the question asked is, 'Yes, but do you think he/she is right?'

Those who are sufficiently literate may benefit from being advised to choose a subject which is uncontroversial within the family such as, perhaps, 'What is the value of a Royal family?' or 'What is your opinion on colour bar/blood sports/capital punishment, etc?' and write down the evidence for and against with the intention of reaching a personal opinion. If the patient objects that he does not know enough about any of these subjects to form any conclusions, it is then pointed out that he does not need to know a lot, no one is infallible on such general topics; the point of the exercise, in fact, is to reach an opinion from the knowledge he already has, and if further information comes to hand at some latter date he may then revise his opinion.

Reserve

People who have been shown no affection in childhood may be unable to show affection to their children, husbands or wives. Where children are concerned it is to be hoped that the other parent can show them affection, while the patient is advised to substitute some other form of activity with them such as playing, singing, or dancing, or reading to them. I believe that this is better, because it is more likely to be acceptable to the child than forced demonstrations of affection.

Where the spouse is concerned, assuming that sexual relations are satisfactory, the problem may be in responding suitably to praise, or to the more casual affectionate greetings, or in showing appreciation for presents and services rendered. A patient who was aware of her deficiencies in this field hit upon the plan of leaving little notes where her husband would find them; when she went to work leaving a meal for him to complete she would write 'I love you' on a card and put it on the tea caddy. But she was still ashamed of her inability to thank him affectionately for presents. She was advised to write him letters in which she expressed her feelings, and thus become practised in expressing feelings when alone, in the hope that this would, in due course, facilitate verbal expression.

Relaxation

Nursing staff give training in this and patients are advised to practise it when fear occurs. The method used is that of Martin.

THERAPISTS

A therapist needs a good self-knowledge. Some have it through natural honesty and insight, others gain it through treatment for neurosis.

Selected ex-patients make good therapists if they volunteer for training; their talent for teaching will have been noticed in tutorials.

The need for therapists to experience and recognize apparently irrational fears in themselves has been discussed under Reassurance (page 41). Admitting hysterical symptoms can be more difficult, but who has not, at some time, made more of a scene than was necessary, or more fuss than was needed about an illness? And the insistence on isolated and unimportant matters of routine can be observed in the most untidy and apparently unobsessional people. The use of alcohol as an occasional sedative is very common. Thus the requirements for understanding neuroses through self-knowledge are present in anyone with enough honesty and insight.

Rebellion

Recollections of childhood conditioning which is still influencing adult behaviour will convince the therapist of the potency of early conditioning. The experiences recalled need not be traumatic and the resulting influences may be desirable, but he can still appreciate the difficulty he would have in breaking such habits.

Recollections of his adolescent rebellions against authority, and the effect these had on his maturing, can enable him to understand the plight of the patient who was too inhibited to rebel. He can then appreciate the current need for such a patient to rebel, accept rebellion with pleasure and satisfaction if it is directed against himself, or explain it reassuringly when a patient describes rebellious episodes at home or at work. On occasions he may even encourage it.

Some therapists find it difficult to accept verbally aggressive rebellious behaviour in patients under treatment for neurosis, and may mistakenly apply the label 'personality disorder' when it occurs. Or if patient rebellion appears to threaten a parent the therapist may see the parent primarily as a supporting figure. He may then discourage the rebellion fearing that parental rejection will harm the patient. In fact, in the case of a patient who has been overdominated in childhood and failed to rebel since, rebellion is an essential component of the bridge to recovery. So it is vital for a therapist to appreciate the value to himself of his own adolescent rebelliousness. I stress this because such recollections are sometimes regretted on account of the distress they may have caused to beloved parents. They should, of course, be seen as part of the normal process of maturing, and one of the inevitable burdens of parenthood.

Detachment

Therapists need to be capable of detachment so that they remain emotionally uninvolved with their patients. Thus, they do not provide the emotional support which the patient seeks, but help him to make a relationship devoid of it. The patient can then begin to understand that he is capable of emotional self-sufficiency. Admittedly most people like being loved but, once grown up, do not need to be and the less we need love the less likely we are to kill it.

In order to attain such detachment it is necessary to have learned to accept unavoidable suffering for oneself and others. But when actually treating a patient it is of primary importance to take up the stance of the cat with one kitten – the interests of the kitten are paramount but the mother cat stands no nonsense. No therapist can successfully treat a patient he dislikes, and if this occurs the patient should be transferred to another therapist. Patients should enjoy the same option.

Popular misconceptions about neurosis

The theory and method of treating neurosis described above is very simple as compared with analytical theory and method. But aspirant therapists should first reject some popular beliefs concerning neurosis and thus bring an open mind to the task.

Fearful people find benefit from facing stressful situations in small doses; doing so will not, as is popularly supposed, make them worse. The patient with a poor self-image will not benefit by having his faults pointed out by fellow members of a group. A display of emotion, if properly understood, can teach the subject something about himself. Through loss of temper he may learn that he can assert himself without the roof falling on his head. Self-abreaction would be lifeless without the emotional content, but it is the subsequent intellectual assessment which is of value to the patient.

The neurotic does not suffer from neurosis because he likes it. This calumny probably arises from the phenomenon of secondary gain in hysteria; it is rarely appreciated that the hysteric would prefer primary gain if he saw a way of getting it. Teaching neurotics methods of solving their problems that they did not learn in childhood is no more likely to make them dependent than teaching the illiterate to read. On the contrary, they will learn the skill and practise it, thus becoming more independent. Explaining neurosis to neurotics, whether in general or personal terms, will not make them resistant to recovery provided they are constantly reassured as to the absence of criticism.

Neurosis is *not* synonymous with inadequate personality. If I define an inadequate person as one who, though sane and of normal intelligence, is *congenitally* incapable of coping with ordinary life, then I greatly doubt his or her existence. The therapist who regards his neurotic patients as inadequate is using a good excuse for failing to treat them adequately. He will be liable to talk down to them and 'temper the wind to the shorn lamb'. Thus he will certainly fail. To succeed a therapist must at least pay his patients the compliment of treating them as his equals in personality.

The sort of do-gooder who believes that anyone who batters a child only does so as 'a cry for help', and who suffers a burning zeal to give that help, will not make a tutorial therapist. It is in part because the method is tough that is succeeds. The therapist needs to be a realist who knows that people are not angels and life is hard; but that pleasure, adventure, satisfaction and fun can be derived from being tough enough to take it.

Aspiring therapists may be held back because they feel a lack of experience. They feel they haven't enough to offer and may not know how to answer their patients. To these I say that it is neither necessary nor desirable to know all the answers because to say, 'I don't know, let us try to work it out together', and then doing so, is more beneficial.

Though perhaps not succeeding brilliantly, the therapist is getting by in life; the patient is not. So it follows that the therapist stands a good chance of teaching the patient something of how to get by. Diffident therapists should bear in mind that they are unlikely to be worse than the psychotherapeutic nothing which is the alternative for the great majority of patients.

4

Communication

Without communication there is no psychotherapy.

LANGUAGE

All teachers should realize that it is essential to use language which is easily understood by all, and when teaching neurotics to bear in mind that pupils are usually too shy to ask the meaning of a word or phrase. Reducing subtle and complex matters to simple terms is not an easy skill, but one without which the therapist will fail. (I often remember my father's head carter who always referred to the 'disc harrows' as the 'dish harrows', by the alteration of one letter changing the unfamiliar into the familiar while remaining equally descriptive. I strive to emulate him.)

The principle of simplicity in language and explanation is of the first importance, and biblical parables provide a good model. Thus, 'You are the family scapegoat, the recipient of the aggression of all of them', is far better expressed as 'They have a lot of anger which they want to get rid of, they know you won't answer back so they pour it on to you'. Use familiar words, mostly of one syllable, be prepared to repeat again and again slowly using different words mostly of one syllable. A parable such as the following is of use: 'If you had three dogs and one of them was an old dog without any teeth left, when you put down their three dinners the two young ones would gobble theirs, and then set on the old dog to drive him off so that they could eat his dinner too. So what you need is some teeth, isn't it?' The teacher can discuss the point of the parable which is: if the patient has (metaphorically) no teeth it is because he fears that, if he showed them, no-one would love him, therefore buying love never pays, so it is better to stand on one's own feet; this takes courage, of which the patient has plenty if he will allow and encourage himself to use it in these conditions.

SOME USEFUL ILLUSTRATIONS AS ANALOGIES

Section through a tree

As many neurotic patients believe that they are either mad or sub-standard humans, to reassure them of the inaccuracy of these thoughts I draw the following:

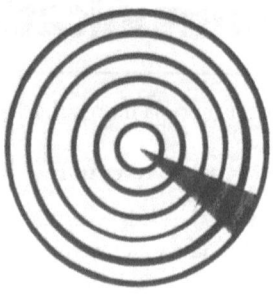

I equate the tree with the person and the shaded segment with the neurosis, which I describe as a small part that as a result of early training error, has not grown up, in other words, is still infantile. Although a very small part of the person it cuts through every ring of growth and runs the whole length of the tree, which is why it causes such havoc in the patient's life; with help, however, the patient can retrain himself so that this segment will 'grow up.'

The glass of water

I use this analogy to explain the way in which painful or shameful memories and past associations cause disturbance in the present, and

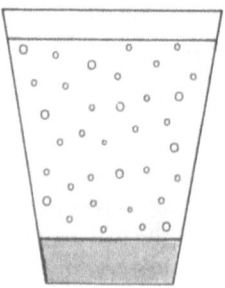

will continue to do so until the patient has reconsidered them in the light of his adult intellectual and emotional development.

I take a glass, fill it from a pond and stand it to settle. This I equate with the mind. The sediment contains minute living plants and animals; these are the memories. The clear water is our conscious mind of which we are aware as we go about our daily rounds. The living creatures give off gases which rise through the water as bubbles; thus the memories and associations disturb our minds.*

Fear and the chest cavity

When frightened our stomach muscles tense into a stiff board, so that if we are struck below the belt we cannot be winded or made helpless. Tensing our stomach muscles pushes up the guts and so reduces the chest cavity; the ribs are held rigid. The diaphragm, a sheet of muscle, is pushed up by the guts from position A to position B (in the diagram) and we prevent it from moving down again as we breathe by pulling in our stomach muscles.

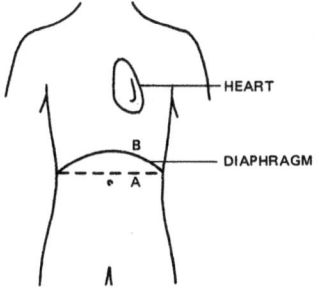

Breathing is then like blowing a balloon up inside a tin can, so we get very little air in our lungs and complain of being breathless. When we force air into this confined space it squeezes the heart, which may upset its rhythm, so we get palpitations or a very fast heartbeat (if the sufferer relaxes when this happens, takes a deep breath into his stomach and coughs, his heart will probably beat normally again).

As a result of this tension around the chest little oxygen is passing through the lungs. Chest constriction hampers the heart which is then able to pump less blood, causing a minor shortage of oxygen to the brain, which may result in dizziness or fainting. If we lie down and relax, however, everything swiftly returns to normal.

*   I think I borrowed this from Leslie Weatherhead and paraphrased it.

Man is an animal

Like the dog, the small child is an emotional and instinctive creature whose ability to think logically has not developed fully. So, like the dog, he learns the difference between good and bad only by connecting good with pleasure and bad with displeasure. He is, of course, entirely dependent on others, initially on his mother and then on his father. If his parents, especially his mother, do not seem to like him it is very likely that he fears for his life as would any young wild animal which would starve if its mother did not want it.

It is easier for us to understand ourselves if we accept our animal natures, because we then accept our angers, jealousies and hates instead of pretending they do not exist, and this makes it easier to control their effects. It is no more wrong to hate than it is to love, and neither are wrong because we cannot help them; promiscuity, however, *is* wrong because it comes from uncontrolled loving, as is murder because it comes from uncontrolled hating.

Man's brain is not basically different from that of other mammals and, like theirs, has developed from the brain of much lower animals (see diagram below): (1) this is the earthworms brain; (2) the dog has added this to the earthworm's brain; (3) Man has added this to both the earthworm's and the dog's brain. We are thus still carrying around the mental equipment of our animal ancestors; all that *we* have done is to add on a piece which makes us think logically and use language. So, basically we are still animals (with an extra piece), and therefore

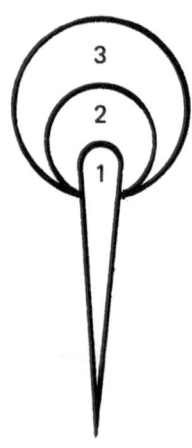

cannot escape from the instincts and emotions which play a great part in our training for life in early childhood before the extra piece is fully developed. When it *is* fully developed we can use our intellects to retrain our irrational emotional reactions.

The only child

Question 'What is the important difference between pictures (1) and (2)?

Answer All children are inferior to adults; they are helpless little parasites. We all tend to get into the habit of feeling inferior and many never get over this habit which is reinforced by competitive work and play at school. In the picture (1) the child has no peers so he feels more inferior and helpless than the children in picture (2) who have peers or near-peers.

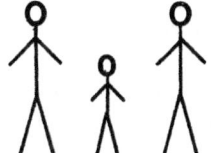 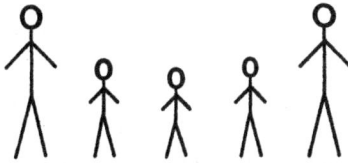

STORIES AS ANALOGIES

The princess and the pea

I tell this traditional fairy story to a patient who is taking pleasure in making more fuss than is necessary; he takes pride in his 'sensitivity', and in this he is compensating for his inferiority feelings by believing himself to be better than anyone else.

Once upon a time there was a prince who was looking for the most delicate and sensitive princess in the world to marry. He must have been rather silly to want this because such a young lady would be likely to complain a lot.

The first princess he found was invited to stay in his castle. The beds in those days were wooden shelves with thick feather quilts for mattresses. The prince ordered a dried pea to be placed under the princess' quilt mattress. The next morning he asked how she had slept. 'Terribly,' she replied, 'There was something about the bed which kept me awake all night.' On the second night the prince ordered that she should sleep on two quilts with the dried pea under them. The next morning the princess came to breakfast smiling, having slept well, so the prince rejected her, sent her home, and invited the next princess to stay. He continued his search until he found a princess who was kept awake by a dried pea under six quilts, and married her.

The three-legged boxer dog

This true story I tell to illustrate tolerance of disability, and point out that many humans allow their disabilities to handicap them far more than is necessary, partly through their expectations, but partly because the disability is a socially acceptable excuse for failure and an apparently adequate reason for not attempting to live life fully. Those with a sense of inferiority expect to fail, and so are most liable to make the most of their physical or mental disabilities, thus spoiling their own lives. I point to Douglas Bader as an example of how exceptional difficulties have been overcome.

The vet's surgery stood on a main road. One day a policeman carried in a boxer puppy that had been run over. One back leg was shattered beyond hope of recovery and the vet amputated it at once. The owner asked the vet to destroy the puppy because he did not want a mutilated dog. But the vet kept the puppy for his children, one of whom was an 8-year-old boy. The puppy grew into a fine specimen, very active on its three legs. The boy was a keen roller-skater on the main road which sloped gently for half a mile. For several years it was common, as one drove along that road, to see the boy roller-skating down the slope, followed by his dog galloping behind wearing a harness. At the bottom of the hill the boy would grasp the harness and the dog would canter back up the hill towing the boy. A good time wasobviously had by all!

How many humans possessed if only three limbs instead of four would make it an excuse for never enjoying themselves in physical activities? The dog, of course, never compared himself with other dogs on four legs, he just enjoyed the three legs he had got.

The old lady and the spaniel bitch

The old lady had never had a dog before though she lived on a farm;

but when her children had all grown up and left home she was sometimes lonely, especially with her husband being out for long hours on the farm, so I housetrained a spaniel bitch and gave it her. She and the bitch became very fond of each other, but sometimes the latter would slip off to hunt rabbits on the farm land.

One day I called to see the old lady and found her in floods of tears – her bitch was away hunting rabbits. I tried to reassure her that the bitch would come to no harm and would return; that, however, was not the problem. 'If she loved me she wouldn't go hunting', she said (she had been an orphan from birth).

I tell this story first to patients whose parents were possessive, and then to those who are possessive of their children. It illustrates well the unreasoning, illogical nature of possessiveness born of emotional insecurity – the old lady evidently felt that her bitch's affection for her mistress could and should be more powerful than a dog's hunting instinct. It also illustrates the futility of attempting to frustrate a natural instinct. I say to parents worried about their children, 'Let them go and they will come back to you; hold on to them and you will lose them for good'.

I have found that such analogies are more easily assimilated if the illustration involves an animal rather than a person.

'Fear and be slain'

This story is about a woman who had recently lost her husband in a car smash; all the children, bar one, were grown up or nearly so, but her youngest child, a boy about 3 years old, was the apple of her eye.

They lived on a main road so she was perpetually anxious about the child's road sense; consequently his curb drill was at least thorough and probably overdone, especially in view of his age.

One day he was walking on the pavement holding hands with a much older child. He broke away, dashed into the road and was instantly killed. His action was apparently impulsive and occurred for no known reason. It seems likely that he was rebelling against over-discipline and nagging on the subject of road safety.

I use this story to illustrate the fact that by trying too hard to avert disaster we actually invite it. I suggest that if we accept the possibility of disaster, face up to the worst that may happen and resolve to endure it if we must, our avoidance techniques will then be more sensible and thus more effective. But if we stand with clenched firsts glaring at the future and saying 'IT MUST NOT happen, I will not allow it to', our avoidance techniques lack common sense.

The fox without a tail

This is a fable paraphrased. The foxes were having a party in the light of the full moon. A latecomer arrived, preening himself on his appearance and showing everyone that his tail was gone. 'Isn't it smart', he said, 'this new fashion is all the rage?' But the foxes laughed; they knew the fool had lost it in a trap.

I tell this story to the patient without confidence tormented by a critical, jealous relative or friend, who is perhaps trying to persuade her that she should do something uncharacteristic like beat her child, leave her husband or persuade him that he should leave his job or sell the house. I point out that the criticizer may be trying to bring the patient down to his/her own 'tailless' level.

The sheep with wanderlust

Sheep usually cling to the flock but there is an occasional independent one. I once had a particularly eccentric sheep which, as soon as her lambs could run, would break through any fence to take both herself and them on expeditions. I have fetched her back as much as ten miles. The point I am making with this story is that we all have a right to our eccentricities as long as they do no harm to others. Of course others will talk and scoff but we don't need to pay attention to that, they've got to have something to gossip about.

Cows in the field, cats in the barn

Take as an example a herd of cows grazing in a meadow, all eating the same grass, drinking the same water, sitting in the same sun or rain. One gives 22 litres of milk a day, while another gives 4 litres; the cows don't care, they aren't worried about which is the best cow among them. But the farmer cares; so it is only humans who compare themselves and worry about being better than their peers.

Or if we take the cat rearing her litter in the barn: she plays with them, they play with each other and learn hunting techniques. Competition and comparison are not needed to persuade them, when the time comes, to go out and catch mice because their built-in drive and pleasure in life will do that. Neither is it necessary for humans to think in terms of success/failure and superiority/inferiority in order to provide the drive to work and play; in fact, such thinking is so much of a handicap that it causes anxiety. So never do what you don't want to do. Sometimes when I wake I don't want to go to work. First I ask whether, if I were going shooting I would feel well enough to do so, if the answer is 'Yes' I then ask myself which I want least, to get up and go or to telephone making excuses and leave someone else to clear up the mess. Hitherto the answer has always been in favour of getting up and going: but tomorrow it might not be so. Thus I retain the freedom to do what I want.

We all do many things we dislike, but we don't have to do things we don't want to do. It is a fact of life that we never do anything well unless we want to do it. To explain further: a patient may say, 'I hate washing up, but it's got to be done!' I reply, 'It's a matter of which you dislike more, to wash up or to live in a clutter of dirty dishes, and put dirty plates on the table for a meal.

The costermonger's pony, or making the best of yourself

We are all a mixture of good, bad and indifferent. We are all thus making the best of a bad job, more so if we don't try to make a silk purse out of a sow's ear, but concentrate instead on happily using our assets to best advantage rather than dwelling regretfully on our weaknesses, which is the usual habit of those with feelings of inferiority.

Many London barrow-boys (costermongers) have a pony and flat cart. Every morning early they go to Covent Garden market at Nine Elms to buy vegetables, fruit and flowers, then drive to their market 'stands' where they sell them.

Take one costermonger with an old slow pony: he *might* complain of this pony because it soon gets tired and can never go faster, or he might congratulate himself on his good fortune at having such a quiet, sensible old pony that stands still all day in a busy, crowded, noisy main street in the centre of town.

Take another costermonger with a young, fast, sprightly pony. *He* might complain of his pony because it won't stand still until it's tired, or he can congratulate himself on having a fast, strong pony which takes him out to the suburbs quickly where he can catch the early shoppers in the main street, while the pony stands getting its breath back. He can then spend the rest of the day driving around selling from house to house. His fast pony will still get him home in time for tea and be fit to repeat it all again tomorrow.

The point of this story is that if one takes a pride in one's assets and makes the best of them, rather than dwelling miserably on one's faults and failings, one's happiness and potential must increase.

The labrador retriever with hysterical conversion

I use this true story to explain the nature of hysterical conversion for those who have it. It also provides a good example of the trigger or precipitating factor of a neurotic symptom.

In the United States a man brought his young labrador to a professional gundog trainer saying that it was useless, unmanageable, and apparently lacked any instincts to do its work. He asked the trainer to have it destroyed. The trainer agreed and put the young dog in a kennel which faced the yard in which he gave dogs their early lessons. For some reason the trainer left the young dog awaiting execution for some days, and then noticed him taking an interest in the dogs he was teaching; when he took the labrador out and started training, the dog responded.

His training completed, the labrador was ultimately sold to a friend of mine who found the dog brilliant both as a gundog and in competitive work. But he had one peculiarity — when a good retriever is sent to retrieve it goes at full gallop, but if for some reason the dog was given the command to stop its left back leg would go into full flexion and become immobile. The dog, too, would become immobile, though dogs are very capable of running on three legs. Gradually, as the years passed, these episodes became less frequent until they ceased when the labrador was about 8 years old.

When my friend had kept the labrador for a few years he happened to meet the woman who had originally bred the dog and at whose kennels the first attempt to train it was made. Although he showed her the dog and its papers he at first had difficulty convincing her that it was the same dog she had rejected. When my friend questioned her on the training methods she had used he found, as he had expected, that the labrador as a keen young dog had been hard to stop when at full gallop. So she had used the 'electric collar', an unpleasant device, which enables a trainer to give a dog an electric shock at a distance, immediately following the command to stop. The labrador's instant response to this overharsh treatment was an inability to absorb any training, so he was rejected as untrainable. Even when he could accept a more gentle training the Pavlovian conditioned reflex was retained — when stopped, that is, frustrated when in pursuit of a desired object, his system reacted as if he had received an electric shock.

As far as I know the electric collar is used only in the United States and even there many trainers reject it. It seems probable that the labrador was galloping when he received the electric shock so only his left paw was was in contact with the ground, and the current earthed through this leg causing the reflex that lasted for so many years.

The rope on the pavement

I tell this story to illustrate the sort of very minor episode which, by association of ideas, can spark off a panic attack or other fear symptoms.

Although I had recovered sufficiently from my neurosis to live comfortably and normally I still suffered symptoms of fear occasionally when in no danger. One day, under no pressure, I was happily waiting at a bus-stop when I became aware of minor symptoms of panic. I coped with the symptoms as, of course, I well could and then looked around to see what had caused them. A few yards away an untidy heap of rope had dropped from a scaffolding. The ridiculous urge to go at once and coil it down tidily told me that this rope was the source of my panic. I had been aware of its presence and, on a subconscious plane, it had set off a conditioned reflex from over 20 years previously.

My father was a keen yachtsman and when he took his children yachting we acted as crew. I was often in trouble for failing to coil ropes the right way; at 8 years old I couldn't master this art and my father set a very high standard. I greatly feared his anger, and 20 years later the subconscious memory still produced panic symptoms in me.

Chased by a bull

When a patient is anxious because his concentration is often very poor, he may believe that his memory is failing. A few simple tests of memory and concentration help to reassure him, but he still asks 'Why?' I tell him that, when frightened, we concentrate on fight or flight but on nothing else, adding 'If you had just been chased by a bull and escaped over the gate, and I asked you what flowers had been growing in the bull's field you wouldn't be able to tell me'.

Looking at an iceberg

To patients who agonize over their sense of inferiority and compare themselves unfavourably with others I say, 'Looking at someone else is like looking at an iceberg, one-tenth above the water, nine-tenths below; you will never know enough about the nine-tenths to discover whether you are better or worse than anyone else. Comparisons are not only odious but pointless.'

Peeling an onion

To the patient who has made good progress, has felt much better, but is regressing again and consequently discouraged, I say, 'The process of recovery is like peeling an onion; you sorted out one problem — the first skin — now you have found the second skin. There is always another skin underneath, but it is smaller than the last one. We have taught and are teaching you to peel your onion. Soon you won't need our help any more, you will know how to peel your own onion by yourself; you will be your own psychotherapist.'

Tom and the guinea-pigs

Tom was head carter on a farm before the days of tractors. An important part of his work was to break in cart colts to prepare them for sale. I often saw Tom handling a rough colt. The great brute might be standing on its back legs waving its front feet around Tom's head while he, quite unmoved, checked and soothed it.

One Sunday the farmer and his wife were walking round the farm when they found that their small daughter's guinea-pigs had escaped from their cage, and were therefore at considerable risk from the farm cats. They had started to catch the guinea-pigs when they saw Tom.

The farmer called out, 'Hey Tom, lend us a hand to catch these dratted guinea-pigs'.

'No Zur!' said Tom backing away 'No Zur! I be afeared o' they, them boites!'

There are, of course, many different kinds of courage. One could hardly describe Tom as a coward any more than a patient with a phobia should describe himself as a coward. What he must learn is to use the courage he has in these conditions.

5

The History and Introduction of the Patient

TAKING A DETAILED HISTORY

Current symptoms

At a first individual interview I take a detailed history beginning with the current symptoms. The patient may be diffident about these; for example, he may complain of headaches or nausea, feeling these to be respectable symptoms (these, of course, must be fully investigated, but that has usually been done). Questioning, without prompting, may elicit the full range of symptoms of anxiety neurosis, obsessionalism or hysteria.

I ask, 'How do you sleep?' and may hear that he can't drop off to sleep at night or wake up in the mornings. I then explain that this is because he does his worrying in bed – as bed is usually the only place in which a child enjoys privacy we are all liable to have developed this habit. I advise him to set aside a time in the day for worrying, to do it with a paper and pencil thus trying to reach positive conclusions, and when he goes to bed to tell himself that he thought about his problem today, and will tomorrow, but not now. I assure him that, with persistence, he will break this habit, and advise him to read in bed.

I ask a patient how he feels in a crowd, at a party, in the street and on public transport. If I elicit anxiety symptoms I ask whether he feels better in the dark; if the answer is 'Yes' I explain that it is criticism that he fears. I ask what he thinks is causing his headaches/nausea and may uncover a rich fantasy of suffering, perhaps, a brain tumour or stomach cancer.

I ask whether he is tidy and likes 'a place for everything and everything in its place' and, pursuing this theme, may hear of obsessional rituals bordering on disablement. During this it is important to 'cap' his stories; if he describes nausea, sweating and giddiness on social occasions I say 'I expect you feel you'd like to sink through the floor and run out of the door, but you don't because you are afraid of making a fool of yourself'. A few such remarks will lead the patient to say, 'You understand!' To which I reply 'Yes, I understand because I've done it myself; I got over it, and you will so don't worry'. If I am then asked, 'After you got over it did it come back?' I answer, 'No, when you have learned to manage it you will always know how to do so'.

My next questions are designed to eliminate a psychotic diagnosis, with special reference to pseudoneurotic schizophrenia in the teens and early 20s and involutional endogenous depression.

CURRENT HISTORY

I then take a detailed history of the events and influences prevailing within the year preceding the onset of the symptoms, and the events anticipated by the patient at the time of the onset. I might record, 'Patient's mother died 9 months before onset', or 'Patient expecting her unmarried daughter to get pregnant at the time of onset', and mentally note that both might appear to the patient as either the loss of a prop or as guilt.

The duration of individual symptoms is recorded. The patient may have always been a worrier, though he may or may not know why. More disabling symptoms may have occurred *de novo* recently or may have recurred. Previous episodes may have presented with different symptomatology. He may have been treated previously by his family doctor or in a psychiatric unit; a 10-year history of taking minor tranquillisers or antidepressants is not uncommon. Enuresis, rejection of school, anorexia, minor hysterical conversions or other neurotic symptoms may have occurred during childhood or the teens without necessarily continuing or recurring.

If the patient has received a course of psychiatric treatment previously I know that prolonged treatment may be necessary. Perhaps this is because he has difficulty in responding to treatment, or maybe previous methods have conditioned him to remain passive while relying on the therapist to cure him, in which case it may take him time to start treating himself.

Previous health

Here I may elicit information concerning childhood, such as periods of separation from parents, traumatic medical or dental episodes, parental rejection of a chronically sick child, the severe sense of inferiority suffered by the physically handicapped schoolchild. Training in hypochondriasis may occur in the child who fears school, in the child of the fussy, possessive mother, and in the rejected child who thinks he can gain kindly attention only by being ill. An adult may be tied to a monotonous job for which his intelligence is too high, through interruption of schooling, or as a result of a child being so frightened of authority that he can not concentrate in the presence of a teacher.

Family history

'Family history', besides offering clues with regard to psychosis, psychopathy and alcoholism, may reveal the reason for a disturbed childhood in a patient who has not inherited these conditions; or there may have been a subnormal sibling with a very strong influence on the patient's childhood. Neurotic parents teach their children social anxieties directly and by imitation, so a question like 'Was your mother one who worried much about what the neighbours thought?' is worth asking.

Childhood history

When taking a childhood history I look for events of which the pre-cipitating factor of the present illness was an emotional repetition. For example, the rejected, much-criticized small girl, when grown, will be likely to fail to respond positively to her young husband's criticism. Instead she will constantly strive to please him, and he may well trade on this. If and when failures build up she may experience panic attacks because a second failure in a close relationship leads her to see herself as a hopelessly deficient person. Though she is unaware that the first failure was no fault of hers, as a result of it her training for life is deficient in managing relationships. A patient who was dragged screaming from her alcoholic mother's arms at the age of 3, to be reared in an orphanage where she was kindly treated and happy, became housebound and remained so for 25 years as a result of her first child, aged 3, being lost in a forest. Although she found him, playing happily, after searching all day the early loss of her mother had conditioned her to respond with chronic fear when forced to face the ever-present possibility of losing her child.

The comments of a schoolteacher, Mr Keningham, (Chapter 10, page 130) give striking examples of the links between early training and neurotic symptoms occurring *de novo* more than 20 years later.

Many patients say, 'But I had a wonderful childhood'. Contrary to popular belief the fact of having been a happy child does not preclude training errors. Those who were miserable are likely to have acquired more unrealistic attitudes of mind, but it is doubtful that anyone gets through childhood without collecting some, and whether or not these cause trouble depends on circumstance (see Chapter 9, patient 3, page 120). And parents have a natural tendency to 'persuade' their children into believing that they are very lucky, perhaps because they have above-average material benefits. So training errors may only be found through detailed enquiry. In order to get at the truth it is often important to reassure patients that no blame is attached to their parents. The questions I always ask are:

'Did your parents get on well?' This may also elicit answers such as 'I never knew my father', or 'My grandmother brought me up', so an outline sketch of the circumstances and the reasons for them can be recorded.

'Did they fight or only shout at each other?'

'Do you remember being frightened when they quarrelled?'

'What did they quarrel about?' The answer is usually money, drink, unfaithfulness or the children, in the last case arousing guilt.

'Whom did you like best, father or mother?' and 'Why?'

'Were you frightened of mother/father?'

'Did she/he hit you much?'

'Were you the cause of the marriage?' This may be worth asking in the case of the firstborn.

I have thus elicited whether or not there was a good parent/child relationship with either parent or both. If the relationship appears to have been at least moderately good with both parents, I start thinking in terms of overpossessive, overexpectant, overindulgent or over-anxious parents, so I ask 'What sort of parents were they?' and persuade the patient to talk round this until the picture becomes clear.

'Were any other grown-ups important in your childhood?' This question elicits information about grandparents, who may have been the child's sheet anchor, the incestuous uncle, the callous childminder or grown-up siblings who may have been spoiling, bullying, or ordinarily kind.

'How many brothers and sisters have you, and what are their ages in relation to yourself?' 'How did you get on with them?' These questions tell me whether the patient was an only child, in fact or in effect. Intense jealousies between siblings suggests either favouritism within the family or a lack of affection throughout, so discussion will elicit which, if either. If neither, was the patient or sibling a bully? The oldest daughter is likely to have had too much responsibility too soon and, in a large family, probably bullied the youngest child. Too much success is often expected of the eldest son; he is also likely to be mother's favourite and thus arouse father's jealousy, and may react by bullying the younger children.

School history

I ask 'At what age did you start school?' 'Were you happy?' 'Did you have plenty of friends?' 'Did you enjoy games?' 'Did you pass any exams?' The child inhibited before he goes to school often suffers further inhibition at school because he lacks the initiative to speak up in class. He is somewhat frightened of the teachers and presents to his peers as one who can be bullied with impunity. The child rejected by his family is likely to seek a family at school, thus making one or two close friends rather than being 'one of the crowd'. The child who feels no-one will pick him up is afraid to fall and so fears sports. The child with a physical defect or infirmity feels inferior, likewise the fat or skinny, the too large or too small. The child dressed worse than the majority feels ashamed of himself, as does one whose father is in jail or whose mother is a prostitute.

Work record

The patient who left grammar school at the first available opportunity is likely to be employed below his mental capacity unless he studied at night school. So he may be bored and frustrated, and may or may not change his job frequently on this account.

Schizophrenics and psychopaths are commonly job-changers, but so are some neurotics. The reason for much changing is important in this context. The neurotic who changes jobs frequently usually does so because he is frightened of foremen and bosses. Neurotics are frightened of change so seek it only when stimulated by a greater and more immediate fear. Unemployment often results from frequent job-changes or from too many sick notices. Those known to have had psychiatric treatment always find difficulty in getting employment.

Overwork due to fear of criticism for failure is common amongst neurotics and exacerbates symptoms. Women are often in full-time work and run a home for several people.

Sex record

I ask 'Did you have plenty of girlfriends or boyfriends when you were young?' Answers vary:

'I've never had any.' Enquire into homosexual practices; these, however, are rare in my patients; shyness is the usual reason.

'I married my first boyfriend/girlfriend.' Enquire into marriage enforced by pregnancy, the urgent desire to escape from home, and the need for a father/mother figure.

'I had a few/enough/a lot and plenty of fun with them.' Score that as normal.

I ask 'Did you and do you enjoy sex?' Most commonly the answer is unequivocally 'Yes'. When the answer is 'No', one finds those who were sexually assaulted in childhood, the sons of overpossessive mothers, those whose parents were intensely prudish, partially impotent men and their wives, frigid women and their husbands, the spouses of those who either don't wish or don't see the necessity for foreplay prior to the sex act, spouses of the unfaithful, mentally or physically battered spouses, couples who practise withdrawal, or, more or less incompetently, one of the non-medicinal methods of contraception, wives who fear both pregnancy (or further pregnancies), and their husbands.

Where fear of sex is the problem, as in the first three cases mentioned and often in impotence and frigidity, psychotherapy is likely to help.

Where the problem is fear of the spouse and/or, in some sense, hatred born of fear or rejection, psychotherapy may improve the marriage but is unlikely to restore the capacity for sexual pleasure with that partner. Counselling on sex and/or contraception is often very helpful in other cases, or sterilization may be accepted as the obvious answer.

The Dutch cap method of contraception is now rarely advised, but when it is the advice on its use grasped by the patient appears to be to insert it immediately before the husband makes entry. This practice would cool the ardours of rabbits, let alone those of a married couple who have been together long enough to have produced all the children they wish to rear. When a patient tells me that this is ruining his/her sex life I advise that the Dutch cap can be worn continuously except during menstruation, but that it must be removed, washed, lubricated and reinserted daily after bathing or washing.

To the patient whose husband is occasionally unfaithful but who, in other respects, is a good husband, good father, good provider and good sex partner I suggest strongly that 'Worse things happen at sea'. I point out that men who are good in all these respects are so because they like women, so one must expect to take the rough with the smooth. I advise the patient to refuse rigidly to know about episodes of unfaithfulness because, as long as the wife doesn't know, the husband is likely to continue to use discretion and so will not shame her publicly. Because he is unlikely to want to confess his guilt, the wife would be foolish to nag him, or consider divorce. Given time, he is likely to prefer the established home, family and circle of friends to the expense and brouhaha of divorce. I reiterate the old axiom, 'A wise woman always lets her husband have her way.'

The state of the marriage in other respects is recorded, and is often not very happy. The insecurity of the neurotic usually leads to over-dependence on the spouse and to anger or tears if unlimited support is not provided. Alternatively I may be treating 'the worse person', the spouse being more disturbed than the patient and his or her behaviour being the trigger factor in the patient's neurosis. Psychotherapy can considerably improve such marital problems.

Details of children and their ages are recorded, also whether any are disturbed, chronically ill or mentally subnormal. Neurotics of course tend to mismanage their children (as has been discussed under childhood history), so one of the most satisfying results of successful treatment is to hear a parent say, 'He/she used to be such a difficult, tiresome, disobedient child, but now he/she is no trouble and always helping me'.

Background lifestyle

By recording whether the house is owned or rented, whether there is a car, and so on, the level of comfort or poverty is established. Hobbies, interests and dependent relatives, if any, are recorded.

Police record

I take this only when I suspect psychopathy, and then discount motoring offences if few, and/or minor and minor crime in adolescence.

Drugs acquired illegally

Most adolescents have experimented a little with soft drugs and rejected them, so this I discount as being within the normal range. Patients addicted to drugs acquired illegally have never been referred to me to my knowledge; they may, of course, have lied to me and then dropped out of the course.

Alcoholic consumption

If excessive I usually offer admission to hospital for 12 weeks for withdrawal under medication, and then initiate tutorial therapy.

Medication

Any medication prescribed is noted, together with the time the patient has been tranquillized or sedated by the family doctor. I very rarely prescribe psychotropic drugs for neurotics.

Previous records

Psychiatric and general records are reviewed.

EXPLANATION

Having taken the history, worked out where training for life was unrealistic and related that to the trigger factor and the symptoms of which the patient complains, I then explain this pattern to the patient.

I say initially, 'Remember that I haven't a crystal ball on my desk, all I have is some knowledge of how people react, so what I suggest may not fit your case; this you must decide for yourself when you think about it'. After discussion I ask, 'Does that fit?' or 'Does that make sense?' I ask questions to make the patient think before offering my answer, for example, 'Why do you think you hit your wife when you are drunk but not when you are sober?' I say that it is not for me to blame the patient for anything, that is not my job and, with a smile, I add, 'Anyway people in glasshouses shouldn't throw stones'. I point out that if one understands the reason for one's reaction control becomes easier.

The explanation of cause and effect in relation to symptoms often brings immediate relief, and occasionally immediate recovery. A patient said of his first interview, 'It was like opening the curtains, I could see *why*'. Such a reaction is not uncommon. To discover that there is a rational explanation for symptoms reassures the patient that he is not mad and what he has to grapple with is within his comprehension. In some cases the rational explanation makes the illness appear more respectable and less shameful.

There are, of course, some patients who seem unable to grasp, or perhaps to accept the explanation, and these will need it repeated, perhaps a number of times, in tutorials. Some reject it saying, 'But it was such a long time ago'. To these I say, 'If you woke up tomorrow to find you had forgotten how to eat with a knife and fork you'd be surprised, but you learned that at the same age as you learned your habits of mind and you have been using both ever since'. Others reject the explanation because they are quite sure they *are* mad or physically ill; for these patients tutorials are very helpful because they hear others accepting similar explanations for their states. Some are certain that they will never change their habits of mind, saying, 'It's the sort of person that I am', and I reply, 'No-one is born that sort of person, certainly you were trained to be that sort of person but what you learned you can unlearn. We will teach you how'.

A typed copy of the history of each patient is included in the folder of the class he attends for the therapist's use. Confidential material is excluded but, if relevant, is mentioned verbally to the therapist. Case histories are included in Chapter 9.

INTRODUCTION TO THE CLASS

Patients have usually been offered a place in a class at the end of the initial interview where the history was taken. If they express fear at the prospect to a sufficient degree that suggests they will not attend, a further individual session is offered. The availability of individual sessions to patients attending classes is explained in the hope that those who do not settle in a class will come to discuss it so that alternatives may be considered.

Patients are continually entering the classes and being discharged from them, so there are always 'old hands' present to help the newcomers. At his first attendance a patient is introduced by the therapist and welcomed. Confidentiality of what occurs at meetings is stressed. He is advised to be cautious in describing his own treatment to his relatives on the grounds that the day may come when he doesn't want to reveal it, so it might be easier to play on the confidentiality rule from the start. He is advised that if he fails to attend without letting us know an ancillary worker may call at his home. It is explained to him that he will not be expected to speak at his first meeting, but thereafter he will be expected to contribute something, however little and however unrelated to his problems. He may comment on football or a television programme if he wishes but, if the rule that all present should speak were not kept, sometimes no-one at all would speak. He is assured of the therapist's help in speaking. Many patients are shy so the first thing the class may teach them is to initiate speech in a group.

The other patients are asked to introduce themselves by name before speaking so that the new member may identify them. The therapist then asks the class, 'Who wants to begin?' A discussion between the therapist and each 'old' patient present follows while the rest of the class acts as audience, the intention of the therapist being to teach. There is some interpatient conversation; at the end of a therapist–patient discussion the therapist may ask for comments or for the help of other members, perhaps by saying 'I don't seem to be getting this over, can anyone help?' The attitude of the therapist is almost invariably helpful and supportive, and from this the class takes its direction. Sometimes the therapist is called upon to be abrasive, but if the class feels that he has overdone it the members will support the patient against the therapist.

Patients always initiate the subject to be discussed with the therapist, and are repeatedly assured that the class is not a public confessional. They should not discuss anything they wish to keep to themselves, but may discuss it briefly with the class therapist after the class or make a clinic appointment.

At the end of his first attendance the newcomer is asked what he thought of the meeting and whether he wants to come again. Unfortunately the answer is nearly always 'Yes', even when the patient is never seen again!

TEACHING THE PATIENT TO USE THE METHOD

Most patients need help in learning to play their parts in the method. The educational standing of many is inevitably poor and prevarication has often been a lifelong habit of the neurotic. The first thing I teach most patients is to listen to the question and then answer it, so that they do not spend my speaking time thinking of the next thing they want to tell me but *listen* to the question. Of course most patients reach my office in the belief that if they 'Tell all' the doctor's magic wand will solve their problems without effort on their parts. If these attitudes are not corrected the conversation proceeds with the irrelevance of a French exercise, for instance: 'Where is the hat of my uncle?' 'I have the pen of my aunt.' The shoes of the child are here'. I may ask, 'When you were little did your parents get on?' to which the patient replies, 'They are both dead now'. I try again, and the question is answered. Or I may ask, 'Did you enjoy school?', and the patient says, 'I don't get on with my husband very well'. After the third irrelevance I say, 'Look, just try to listen to the question and answer it; if we are to help you this is something you must learn to do because this is how the treatment works. You don't have to answer every time; if you don't want to tell me you only have to say so, or say you don't know *if* you don't know. I'm sure you will do very well if you listen and try to answer'.

In tutorials prevarication also occurs:

Therapist 'How many lampposts have you worked up to?' (see page 78).

Patient 'The weather has been terrible, hasn't it?'
Therapist (With a bright smile) 'How many lampposts have you worked up to?'

Simple logical deduction must also be taught, for example:

Therapist 'A week ago you were quite sure you had heart trouble; you know that we have tested your heart and found it sound. You have done very well in seeing for yourself that you thought you were ill with one thing or another for a long time because you felt you needed attention. You have spent a week on the ward where you have seen some people with mental illnesses, and you now tell me that you think you are mad. Why do you think that?'
Patient 'I don't know, I just feel like it'.
Therapist 'You say you thought you were ill because you needed attention, then what is the likely reason for thinking you are mad?'

When a patient begins treatment he often talks about nothing but his symptoms, endlessly repeating himself. This is because he hopes that the doctor can remove his symptoms and will do so if he knows how terrible they are. He must first be persuaded that he can only cure his symptoms himself, though the therapist will teach him how, and has in fact already started this teaching. Then, through the therapist's repetition of the teaching and kindly insistence thereon, he must be persuaded to concentrate on this positive action. A milestone is passed when a patient who since he started treatment some weeks ago, has always opened his discussion with a woeful description of all that he has endured during the past week, starts instead by recounting with pride the progress he has made in carrying out what he has been taught so far.

6

Fear and Self-esteem

Fear is the universal problem of neurosis so the therapist's first task is to teach the patient to cope with fear and to do so without the use of medication; if he is already use to medication he will only be asked to withdraw this gradually when he has made considerable progress in managing his fear. Or, putting the problem another way, all patients first come to therapy because they want to be rid of their symptoms, which are due to fear, so their co-operation, which is essential, will be more easily obtained if treatment is immediately directed towards coping with the symptoms. It has to be explained, however, that the therapist cannot remove the symptoms; this the patient must do for himself when he has been taught how.

TREATING FEAR

The following eight steps have been found most beneficial.

(1) Take a detailed history at individual interview, explaining cause in childhood training and effect in the occurrence of symptoms in later life. Where in rare cases no cause is found, as in a case of amnesia for childhood, cause and effect are then explained in general terms and the cause often emerges during treatment. Therapist persuasion may be needed because patients are sometimes ashamed to admit the child-hood causes, but when they have done so the sympathy of the class is therapeutic.

(2) Explain, in tutorials or further interviews, the physiological symptoms of fear – that they are incurable, being an important part of

74

our survival kit; that they are uncomfortable, like being cold or hungry; that as a result of tolerating them they reduce in force – but that the effect of running away from them is only to increase the set of circumstances in which they occur. (Thus a man who has his first panic attack on a train thereafter won't travel on trains, but still gets the next attack on a bus, so he buys a car, gets the next attack in the car, so he becomes a pedestrian, gets the next attack in the street so he stays at home, gets the next attack watching television so he stays in bed.) A large part of the fear of panic is fear of making a fool of oneself in public, but other people are usually unaware of one's panic.

(3)   Explain that in each case individual courage has been inhibited under the circumstances in which panic occurs, so the patient has to learn to apply it in these circumstances. He must be assured that his courage *in general* is not in question since he is often prepared to face near-intolerable situations to avoid doing the very action for which his courage is inhibited. He can then see that the task is one of redirecting the courage he possesses. I often ask 'If you were alone on the bank of the canal and saw a child drowning, would you go in after it, whatever your particular fear?'

(4)   Teach the patient to desensitize himself. Advise him to do the thing he fears daily for gradually increasing periods, in effect to seek out fear in order to learn to tolerate it, which is easier to tolerate if the patient has deliberately looked for it of his own volition. Having found fear and tolerated it, for two minutes on the first day, for four minutes on the next, and so on, he should then pat himself on the back as if he had run a tough race. The patient must be warned against tolerating fear for too long, however, because this may reinforce the habit of fear in those circumstances. But it must be stressed that daily exercise of courage for very gradually increased periods is absolutely necessary. The patient should allow himself no excuse, but every time he does what he fears makes it easier to carry out the next time.

(5)   Teach relaxation to those who attend for this and advise patients to use it when frightened.

(6)   Advise the patient never to go into a situation he finds frightening without having prepared a socially acceptable excuse for leaving it; the readiness of the excuse will reduce the likelihood of his needing it.

(7)   Ask 'What were you afraid of?' when a patient says he has suffered fear. On a number of occasions he is likely to answer, 'I don't know'. The causes both in childhood and currently are then rediscussed and re-explained. The patient says 'I don't know', partly because he

has not understood but largely because he does not believe the therapist, when he says that the fear is not the patient's fault, and that he is not a second-class human being. He will, however, believe his fellow patients and see that the causes explained to them by the therapist could also be true of him. What is wrong with him then appears more respectable because it is explicable, and he at last believes that he is no worse than other people.

(8) Explain that even though panic feels as if it would escalate until it drives one mad, in fact this cannot happen because there is a built-in limit to the amount of fear or pain we can feel, rather on the same principle as a thermostat.

TEACHING THE SYMPTOMS OF FEAR

Patients suffering these are likely to believe that they portend lunacy or fatal disease, so a simple explanation is often remarkably curative. I say, 'When we are frightened of something nature prepares us to fight or run away from an animal like ourselves, just as if we still lived in trees or caves as man did many years ago. So the feelings we get when we are afraid are the same as those the dog, cat or horse gets, though we may not get them all at once.

Take the feelings one by one, starting at the top.

(1) Prickly feeling in your head and sometimes down your back as well: this is your hair standing on end to make you look bigger to frighten your enemy. Think of a cat standing up to a dog, its back arched and its top hair on end. By the same principle the Guards wore tall hats in battle to make them look bigger.

(2) You cannot see clearly things close to or far off, but if you hold out your fist you can see that perfectly: that is the distance at which you would need to see your enemy clearly to hit him, so the focus of your eyes is fixed at that distance.

(3) Your muscles tense up ready to fight or run, with the neck muscles being extra tense because if your enemy hit you on the chin when your neck muscles were slack he could break your neck. If you stay frightened for long this may give you a headache so remember your relaxation exercises. Your stomach muscles will also be extra tense because if you were hit in the stomach when they were slack you would be winded, lying on the ground helpless, ready to be attacked. Tense stomach muscles elevate the diaphragm which leaves your heart

too little room to work causing palpitations. You need to breathe down as well as out sideways to stop this, so remember your relaxation exercises, lie on the floor, lay your hand on your stomach and make your breathing move your hand up and down. If you stay frightened for long this may give you a headache, so relaxation is important.

(4)   Your heart goes fast to pump plenty of blood to your brain and muscles so you can think quickly and run or fight.

(5)   Your skin goes cold, so you shiver and sweat because the blood leaves your skin to supply your muscles and brain.

(6)   You will run faster or fight better with empty guts because you will be lighter, so you may feel sick, actually be sick, or empty bladder or bowels.

(7)   All these things happen while, though afraid, we are still able to fight or run away, but sometimes if we are very frightened we become literally paralysed with fear; this could be called nature's anaesthetic – you feel that you can't move, speak or think, or you may curl up in a ball like a hedgehog. When, sometimes frightened people stand bowed they have started a reflex action to curl up.

AGORAPHOBIA

I have only met one true agoraphobic; as a small child, he had been subjected to daylight bombing and machine-gunning and to his mother's natural intense anxiety concerning these hazards.

The many other patients who have been referred under this diagnosis have all feared the adverse opinions of other people, and so were afraid to be in places where they might meet others. They became more afraid the further they got from the privacy of their homes; terrified in situations, including public transport and social gatherings, from which they felt they could not readily escape; liable to cross the road if they saw an acquaintance coming towards them; usually more able to go out in the dark when potential critics could not see them so well, or with someone whom they felt to be answerable for their social acceptability, generally a relative.

Agoraphobics also felt better when doing something which seemed socially estimable, such as pushing a pram, going to work, taking a child to school or the dog for a walk. Their behaviour had often already aroused comment from neighbours (perhaps the husband was doing all the shopping or the wife all the outdoor repair work), so the patient was known to be 'bad with his/her nerves', which exacerbated the symptoms through inferred condemnation.

Such a patient presents a three-fold problem: he must be taught both to manage his symptoms of fear; and to improve his self-concept because his expectation of criticism springs from his poor opinion of himself, and he must learn to manage interpersonal relationships more assertively so that he is confident of his ability to answer back in the event of any criticism.

Managing fear

An agoraphobic is afraid to leave the house, so will not do so until he absolutely must go out, perhaps to shop for essential supplies for the family; he then goes out with the fear of failure added to that of being outside. He is advised first to try and arrange for someone to do any essential shopping for him for a while; and then to find a time in the day when nothing is pressing on him and go to the nearest lamppost outside his house. He should stand there until panic seizes him and then remain at the lamppost tolerating panic for *two* minutes, taking deep breaths and reassuring himself that he is only frightened, a normal experience. He should then go home, praise himself for his courage, and cosset himself in which ever way appeals to him. The next day he should go to the second nearest lamppost and tolerate panic for *four* minutes, on the next day to the third nearest lamppost for *six* minutes, and so on till he can move freely and tolerate panic with equanimity. Panic will then begin to fade because, knowing that he can tolerate it, he also knows that he need not make a fool of himself in the presence of others when panic seizes him. So the patient no longer fears panic and begins to understand that it was his fear of panic which caused it, or at least exacerbated it.

The patient is advised never to resist panic nor try to escape it, but to relax, accept it and let it roll over him as he might lie on a beach and allow a wave to roll over him. Some patients, demonstrating misplaced heroism in the cause of the speedy recovery which they crave, will immediately go forth to endure panic for an hour or more. So when advising patients to endure panic, they must be warned to avoid pro-longed endurance, which only reinforces the habit of fear in that situation, but instead to work up gradually with regard to time and distress.

Patients often ask about medication for panic, and I tell them that if there were any drug which could cure fear it would be prescribed for all the troops in war time. I explain that because fear is an essential piece of our survival kit our systems respond to a drug which reduces the sensations of fear by rapidly getting used to it to keep the survival kit intact – hence habituation and the necessity to increase the dose frequently. I advise patients that they would be wiser to learn to manage fear so that it no longer troubles them unduly, than attempt to smother it temporarily with medication.

To the query whether fear is likely to kill them, I reply that if fear were commonly fatal few troops would reach battles alive.

The principle of the lamppost method is later extended to cover public transport – one stop today, two tomorrow and so on, or shops – one purchase the first day, two the second, or social occasions – ten minutes in the bar or bingo hall tonight, 20 minutes tomorrow. When it comes to social gatherings the patient is advised never to go without having prepared an excuse to leave at will, for instance (looking at a watch), say 'I must just slip out to 'phone my mother/uncle/sister who is ill, I promised I would 'phone at X o'clock. No I won't use your 'phone, it will disturb the party'. If the excuse is needed more than once then the number was engaged the first time. Or a mild enteritis can be invented so that the patient gets a breathing space in the toilet or bathroom as often as desired. The availability of escape greatly reduces the need for it. Patients are advised to get up and leave the tutorial meetings when panic-stricken; but they are urged to return to the situation which caused panic when it has subsided. Attention is drawn to the fact that when one has withdrawn from a fearful situation and become calm the situation no longer looks as fearful as it did before, so this is the ideal moment to face it again; but that if one does not face it again straightaway shame and failure are added to fear so return to the situation inspires horror. To illustrate this: both horse and rider fall at a fence, but if the rider doesn't remount and ride over another fence at once both are liable to suffer a loss of nerve.

The same principle is applied to any fear-invoking situation: a man who feared water transport started by taking a pleasure dinghy out on a lake daily; a man who could not take his car more than a mile from home worked the distance up at the rate of a quarter-mile a day; a woman who could not stand lifts started with going up one floor and walking down; and a woman who feared dogs went visiting a neighbour's dog daily. All these successes, however minor, caused great satisfaction, and progressively overcoming what 'everyone' calls their silliness was invaluable for their self-respect.

INFERIORITY

In teaching improvement of the self-concept I say, 'We are all good at some things and bad at others; you are noticing what you are bad at and taking for granted what you are good at. If you think back you will remember that you were taught to do this in childhood. If you tried to train a dog like that you wouldn't get on very well; if you kicked it and shouted at it when it did wrong, but failed to rub its ears and tell it that it was a good dog when it did right, it would end by cringing at your feet and doing nothing at all. In this matter you need to 'be your own mother', notice what you do well, pat yourself on the back for them, and never miss the chance to tell yourself you have done well.

Are you a good cook, gardener, handyman, needlewoman, cleaner, decorator, car driver? Take a big piece of paper, write your name and the names of four or five friends along the top and down the side, make a list of various activities you all often do. Then give each name marks out of ten for these skills, add them up, and you will find that you are average. I don't think that many patients actually perform this exercise but it can give them a new look at themselves.

I try never to miss a chance of commending a patient. Mrs Jones has passed six lampposts since the last tutorial: 'Well done, that's great, go on like that and you'll be right in no time'. For the first time in his life Mr Black has told his mother he can't do what she wants because he has another engagement: 'Good for you, splendid! And she took it well, didn't she?' I ask Miss Brown a question to which I get a clear and thoughtful answer: 'Top of the class, you are learning fast'.

I explain that an inhibited child goes to school at five with a sense of inferiority, so he boasts, 'My Dad is bigger than yours, our house is bigger than yours, I can run faster than you', and so on. Teacher and classmates jump on him. 'You big-headed little so-and-so'. Thus he learns that he mustn't think well of himself: but the uninhibited child at school has no need to boast, so he is never taught not to think well of himself and does so normally.

When teaching a patient to desensitize himself with regard to his inferiority feelings it is useful to advise him to give up a short time every evening going through the acts and events of the day and mentally listing what he did that was both good and bad. He went to work, she cleaned the house, cooked the meals, shopped and saw to the children, he did a bit in the house or garden in the evening, they both spoke to workmates and neighbours with ordinary courtesy and played with the children. If he/she has had a good day, he/she scores 10 out of 10 for superiority. Perhaps, however, he got angry with his wife for no good reason, or she shouted at the children when they hadn't deserved it, so knocking off two marks for that it's still 8 out of 10.

It might be worth sparing a thought as to why tension mounted to the point of minor explosion; it was probably fear of failure so one has to learn to accept failure. Perhaps he forgot to buy the dog biscuits on his way home, or she put a dish down carelessly and broke it. 'So what? Half a mark off at most, the dog will manage on stale bread and gravy and you can't expect to run a house without breaking something sometimes. Would you think the worse of someone else for such minor accidents? Is it perhaps only you that must never do wrong? Was it when you were a child that you learnt that *you* could never afford to do anything wrong, other people might but you mustn't? Wasn't that just because they didn't like you? Start to like yourself, work at it, if you try you'll find you can do it, all you've got to do is break the bad habit you learnt in childhood of hating yourself. Every time you catch yourself being critical of yourself, stop and think of something you've done well, and every time you catch yourself feeling inferior think of something in which you've succeeded. This is how to use your wits to retain your feelings; you know you aren't bad or inferior, so make what you *know* correct what you *feel*, and you will break the habit'.

To the patient who says, 'But I *am* inferior because I have bad nerves', I reply, 'You've got the cart before the horse, you've got bad nerves because you feel inferior'. Looking at someone else is like looking at an iceberg, one-tenth above the water can be seen, nine-tenths below the water can not be seen. We never know enough about another person to know whether he or she is really better or worse than we are, so we never know whether we are better or worse than anyone. We just have to take it on trust that we are about average on the good/bad scale, and put up with ourselves the best way we can.

To the patient who says, 'I feel so unworthy, I'm not doing anything to help other people', I say, 'If you aren't at work now you have been, and you will be again when you feel better or can get a job. Hospitals, schools, libraries, police and a hundred other things are all supported by industry and commerce. Your job is part of industry so you are doing something very important for other people; without workers like you there would be no public services because there would be no money to pay for them. The tycoon in Manchester making his million and the missionary running a leper colony in the South Seas are both doing an equally good job for mankind and both are doing it for the satisfaction they get out of it, so you can not say that either one is better than the other. The great reformers, like Florence Nightingale, were leaders in their fields, but they didn't create civilization. Thinking back only a few hundred years ago, people were burnt alive for their religious beliefs, or hung in cages outside castle walls and left there for years or until they died. If there was a revolt against the government of the day in a particular area the whole area would be laid waste leaving the guilty, innocent, men, women and children to starve together. We are a lot better off than we were a few hundred years ago. Changes have been effected by millions of ordinary people who did a decent job as well as they could and lived ordinary decent lives, each of them putting a very small brick into the wall against barbarity; if any one of us manages to build in more than one very small brick he will be very lucky'.

To the patient who says, 'I feel so useless because I can't work (or can't get a job)', I say 'When I was a student doing my training in the fever hospital there was a man living in an iron lung, he'd been there a long time, probably years. If it was propped up just right for him he could just turn the pages of a book, but the rest of him was paralysed by polio. Most of the people working in the hospital used to find excuses to go to his ward and have a word with him because he was such a terrific person; he in fact was helping us, we were only keeping *him* alive. No-one with any spirit likes being dependent on other people, so we would rather work; but if we can't work it doesn't mean to say we are useless: 'They also serve who only stand and wait'.

ASSERTION

In a typical session the following interchange might take place.

Therapist If I say to you 'why do you come here in blue trousers and black shoes' what are you going to say to me?

 A deadly hush, deep thought, then.

Patient I'm sorry, Doctor, I haven't got any blue shoes.

Therapist (to the group) Anybody got any other answers?

Chorus (from the old hands) Mind your own bloody business!

Therapist (to patient)   See what I mean? I am your servant, they pay me
to treat you not to insult you.

Thus the therapist uses the authority with which the patients endow
him to devalue authority, and the respect in which they hold him to
teach them not to respect power or position. They will always respect
worth when they meet it.

If the patient says, 'What I'm going to say may sound silly', I reply,
'It won't sound any sillier than plenty of things I've said, so carry on'.
Or if he says, 'I'm so frightened' I say, 'I know just how you feel, I
remember feeling the same, and it's horrible. But if you do what I say
the day will soon come when you will not be frightened of anyone, not if
it were the Devil himself, and that is beautiful!' They say 'You!' and I
say, 'Yes, that's how I know what to say to you'.

If a patient says, 'I have no confidence', I say, 'No-one has any
confidence to do anything until they have done it. The first time you
answer back it's an act of blind courage and you are terrified; but when
you find that the roof hasn't fallen on your head, next time it's easier'.

HYPOCHONDRIASIS

The hypochondriac is an hysteric. For example, we speak loosely of
cancerphobia, which is not a true phobia but a form of hypochondriasis.

To recapitulate briefly what has been said of hysteria in Chapter 1:
In escaping from unpleasant reality the hysteric has learned in childhood to dream – 'If you can dream and not make dreams your master'
– but the hysteric is the slave of his. There are, of course bad as well as
good dreams, so he not only has Walter Mitty-type dreams, but also,
perhaps after a programme on television, dreams that he will commit
murder, is schizophrenic or has cancer. He then suffers severely
because he is very frightened and the physiological symptoms of fear
lend colour to the dream, thus convincing him. Both bad and good
dreams attract limelight so in discussion the therapist should attempt to
dissolve the limelight, and make cancer and death look as ordinary as
they really are.

Hypochondriacs come to me convinced that they have an organic
disease that the doctors have failed to discover and that more penetrating
examination would reveal. Reassurance is worse than useless – offering
it is like trying to fill a bucket with a hole in the bottom; the patient has
an insatiable appetite for it because it is limelight, so reassurance

exacerbates the hypochondriasis. Having told the patient once that investigation shows nothing physically wrong with him I explain that it is not in his imagination but in reality the physical symptoms of fear which cause his suffering, and these I describe in detail. Then there might be the following conversation:

Patient *But I'm sure* there is something wrong.

Therapist If I'm wrong and you are right, and you have something wrong that we can't find, it's the same as having an incurable illness, isn't it? Just the same as having rheumatism, which can't be cured, so you'll have to accept it and put up with it.

Patient So you think I am really ill.

Therapist No, *I* don't think so, *you* do. I think you're frightened, that's all.

Patient But I might die.

Therapist Yes, you might die, we all shall one day; either you or I might be dead on the road on the way home, life's like that.

Patient But I don't want to die.

Therapist Most of us don't, but we have to put up with it.

Patient Then you think I'm going to die?

Therapist Certainly one day, like the rest of us. Accept it, cross the bridge when you get to it; you're alive today, enjoy it. Apply your courage to the task of accepting death, you've plenty of courage so use it.

Patient No, I'm a coward, I'm always frightened of everything.

Therapist Courage isn't a matter of not being frightened, courage is *being* frightened and coping with it – you just haven't learned to use your courage. Next time you get a pain and think you've got cancer just say to yourself, 'I'm not going to make myself miserable over this and I'm not going to make a fuss about it either; if I've got something the doctors can't find and it kills me it will just have to kill me because I've done all I can and so have they. I'm alive today, I'm going to enjoy it.' Then do something that makes you happy, and think how good it is to be alive *today*, never mind tomorrow. Every time you do that it will be easier to do it the next time. Courage improves with practice; it's an enormously valuable asset to have acquired – a skill like swimming or hitting a ball or driving a car – and when you've learned it you'll feel a foot taller.

Patient But, Doctor, these dreadful pains!

Therapist '*Dreadful*' pains! What makes you think your pains are any worse than other people's? You are deliberately exaggerating them in your own mind, that is why you are so frightened of them. Pain hurts much more if you are frightened of it. When you get a pain relax, and make up your mind just to let it happen, then do something you enjoy and you'll forget it.

Patient But I'm so frightened.

Therapist Yes, I know, the fear causes the pain, the pain makes you more frightened and that makes the pain worse. Accept it, put up with it, it's the only way.

At a typical therapy session I ask the class, Who wants to start?

Mrs H I'll start then. I've had a dreadful week because of what you said last time. You said that if a patient couldn't get off tablets at home she'd have to come into hospital to get off them! I went home in a dreadful state, I felt terrible, my heart was pumping, I was crying, I couldn't breathe, I thought I'd be sick. . . . [*carries on in this vein*] When I got home I lay on the floor screaming until my husband promised he wouldn't let me go into hospital; but the next day I was just the same and. . . .

Therapist Stop there a minute. Why did you want your husband to promise that?

Mrs H Because I felt so dreadful, my stomach was. . . .

Therapist Stop there. You know as well as I do that no-one can force you into hospital unless you are suicidal, so why did you want that promise?

Mrs H I felt so dreadful I didn't think. I'm *terrified* of hospitals. I'd die of fright if I went in to one. I've had a dreadful week. My head. . . .

Therapist Supposing you had a car accident, and you were carried in unconscious, do you really think you'd die when you woke up?

Mrs H No, no, perhaps not. But I've had a dreadful week, yesterday I was crying at work and I haven't slept. . . .

Therapist Stop there. You've told us three times that you've had a dreadful week and so on. Why?

Mrs H I don't know. I thought you ought to know.

Therapist (*to class*) Why?

Several patients She wants to punish you.

She wants us to be sorry for her.

She wants attention.

She wants to feel important.

Therapist And why did she ask her husband to make that promise?

Patients   For the same reasons.
Therapist   But why does she want pity, attention and importance?
Patients   She's afraid.
She has no confidence in herself.
She has a poor opinion of herself.
Therapist   Right. She doesn't feel she can cope with life on her own so she is looking for people to support her. So she imagines disasters, such as being dragged screaming into hospital and dying of fright, to make a reason for other people giving her support, though if she thinks she knows quite well that these disasters can't or won't happen.

It's what we'd all do in her shoes, of course, and she's been doing it since she was three years old. Her imagination is her strong point, so it was entirely reasonable and sensible as a small child to use it to escape from unpleasant realities in an unhappy childhood, and equally reasonable to use it to manage other people and so get some of the attention she then needed; but now these habits are making life more difficult, not easier. She is terrifying herself with her imaginings and allowing her dreams to seem more real than reality. Do you get the picture, Mrs H? And do you understand that no-one is criticizing you? If we hadn't been through the same sort of thing ourselves we wouldn't know enough to explain to you what you are doing and why. You see, you are grown-up now, you are very competent, you can manage life without support; but when you were little you couldn't manage, no-one can. Life was made too difficult for you as a small child, so you got into the habit of feeling you couldn't cope and must have support. You still have that habit and it's making your life a mess; *but you can break the habit.* You've spent a miserable week for no real reason at all. Next time something like this happens try to stop and think, 'Is this scene really necessary? What good will it do me? Do I really need attention now I'm grown-up? Surely I can stand on my own feet instead.'

This lesson is likely to need repeating in relation to different episodes, and the urge to blame and punish the therapist needs discussion in terms of transference. In other aspects, however, further treatment is, as for the anxiety state, a matter of teaching self-esteem and the proper uses of courage and agression.

SELF-PITY

This kind of attention seeking is where the patient is paying attention to himself and wallowing in it, so naturally it often spills over into demanding attention of others on account of one's 'misfortunes'. When the habit is well established it destroys the capacity for enjoyment because every event and circumstance is automatically converted into sorrow or misfortune as it passes through the sufferer's mind. For example, 'Did you enjoy yourself in Spain?' 'Well, I suppose I should have: but we all got sunburned and then it was really windy one day so the sand got in the picnic, not that the food was much, they don't know how to make sandwiches and of course we all got stomach upsets. I was glad to get home really'.

The children of such a parent are likely to be at risk because they are seen only as a burden to be nobly borne. When this sentiment is expressed I ask the patient why he or she keeps the children and point out that doing so is voluntary, that many people abandon their children to the care of the state so perhaps the patient should do so. The usual reaction is: 'Oh, no! I couldn't do that'.

When I ask why not I am told that either the patient loves the children or that he/she is too high-minded. If it's a matter of love, I suggest that he/she is lucky to have the children, plenty of people complain bitterly if they can't have any, and every time he/she is finding them burdensome ask: 'Do I really want these kids because I can get rid of them if I don't?'

If it is a case of highmindedness I point out that this is a luxury, no-one is under any compulsion to be high-minded, we are pleasing ourselves in that we derive self-satisfaction out of believing ourselves to be virtuous, so if we do so we should take pleasure in it, and if we can't why do it? The answer is 'But what would other people say?' To this I reply, 'It doesn't matter who you are or what you do, a quarter of the people you mix with will think you're pretty good, another quarter will think you're pretty bad, and half will be too busy with their own affairs to make up their minds one way or the other, so worrying about what other people think is a waste of time'.

When the patient is ready to admit to self-pity I say that it's just a bad habit that can be broken by consciously and deliberately noticing everything which one enjoys – especially all those things which one takes for granted such as a warm room on a cold day, sunshine, going to bed when one is tired, eating when one is hungry, stretching when one wakes up, soaking in a hot bath and so on. I point out that this bad habit is destroying all enjoyment.

A patient who had listened to this teaching said at the next tutorial,

'When I thought about what you said to that lady last week, I saw that was what I was doing too, so I said to myself, 'Snap out of it, time to be miserable when you are dead! I'm feeling much better'.

SUFFERING

Patients sometimes say they feel worse as a result of attending tutorials because they have to listen to other people's troubles and, being sensitive, they suffer too. I say, 'Life is full of suffering, it's going on all the time, we all know that; but have you noticed that we only complain about what we see, as long as we don't see it we pretend it isn't there. Surely what we need is to accept suffering as part of life just as we accept joy?' The answer is to the effect that the patient is too sensitive to do that. I ask what is meant by sensitivity and, getting no answer, say, 'Sensitivity is only awareness, if you are a sensitive person you know what other people are feeling; but you won't be much good to them if you just run away from it. Suffering does good as well as harm, we learn from it, grow through it, and survive – that is experience. Learn to accept it and don't allow yourself to brood on it. Put up with other people's suffering just as you put up with your own. That is one of the things that you come hear to learn to do'.

I also tell them this story: When I lived in the suburbs and kept dogs, strangers would knock on my door and ask 'Please will you take Fido to be put to sleep for me? When I asked 'Why?' they said, 'I couldn't do it myself, I'm much too sensitive', so I asked them why they thought I wasn't! I then told them politely that to send Fido to be put to sleep in the care of a stranger would be unkind, insensitive and cowardly because Fido would be afraid, whereas if its master or mistress took it to the vet, as he or she must have done many times before, mustering the self-control to behave as if it were just another visit, Fido would know nothing about it.

THE STATE OF BEING NEUROTIC

Patients often feel ashamed at needing psychiatric treatment, so I tell them that the word 'neurotic' has a different meaning medically from its colloquial sense and tell them my definition (see Chapter 1, page 18). Most people are at least somewhat neurotic and many are doing a lot of damage because they do not seek treatment when they should.

The handful of young men who seek treatment because they beat up their wives are a very small proportion of wife-beaters; these are behaving responsibly, whereas those who batter and fail to seek treatment are at least equally neurotic *and* irresponsible with it. I tell them that neurotics are people with a high loading of goodwill and advise them how to assert themselves towards those who verbalize scorn towards them.

For patients who often regard themselves as being congenitally second-class human beings because they are neurotic, I draw the diagram of a section through a tree, showing the lines of growth (see Chapter 4, page 50). I say that at present neurosis is interfering with the whole of the patient's life; but when he has learnt, as we shall teach him, to make that very small segment grow to be normal, the whole patient will then be just as normal as any of us. This may not be saying much – what is normal, after all? What society regards as normal varies from century to century and from place to place. Here a man who marries two wives has committed a crime, but in some Eastern countries it is almost expected of him. Are we not all entitled to our odd little ways provided they don't harm other people?

'It's not your fault you are neurotic', I say, 'Why be ashamed of it? You might just as well be ashamed of having measles or a broken leg. If other people are horrible about it they should be ashamed, not you.'

I tell them a story I once read about Winston Churchill. He was in the underground centre of government during the war, a place of long narrow corridors with doors opening into small cells for the inmates. Beside these doors often stood empty milk bottles. One night Churchill, called from his bed to a conference, sleepily set forth down the corridor where he happened to kick over a bottle, and this enraged him. He pursued the bottle down the corridor kicking it as if it were a football till it smashed. I ask, 'If Churchill could on occasions be childishly ridiculous, surely we can too?'

I also tell them that all neurotics are potentially nice people because their inborn factor is goodwill, which is consideration and caring. I explain that this factor caused them to learn in infancy to be so anxious to do and say the right things to please other people at their own expense, and that other people have been trading on it ever since.

TREATMENT FOR NEUROSIS

Some patients are frightened of treatment; they ask whether it is 'brainwashing' or whether it will change their personalities – might Dr Jekyll become Mr Hyde? I assure them that treatment can't change the personality with which we are born, it is unalterable except through major brain disease. To explain what treatment can do I take a botanical analogy: 'The forsythia is a lovely bush which grows yellow flowers in the spring. If you take a young plant of this bush you can train it to grow up a trellis, as ivy grows up a wall, but you have to tie the twigs onto the trellis, or you can plant it in the open and let it grow into its natural shape. If you took an old bush grown in its natural shape you would not be able to train it onto a trellis because the branches would be too tough to bend the way you wanted; if you forced it onto the trellis it would soon break the bonds or the trellis. This is all that 'brain-washing' can do, the effects only last a few days (when the Russians use it on someone they wish to condemn in a trial, they have to arrange the trial at once, as soon as the brainwashing has taken effect, because it wears off quickly and cannot be repeated). However, with any forsythia plant that has been grown on a trellis, if you cut the bonds and removed the trellis, the plant would grow to its natural shape; this is psycho-therapy – we teach you to cut the bonds and you can do your own growing.

SHYNESS

Patients complain that they can't make conversation, that everything they say sounds silly. I say, 'Have you ever listened to what people say at a party or in a pub? If you do you'll find that it nearly all sounds silly, it's not meant to be clever, people are just making friendly noises like a lot of starlings chattering on a telegraph wire'. We then play a game to teach them to make conversation: the first one in the circle says a word, his/her neighbour says the first word that the previous word reminds him of, and so on all round the circle, for example: Horse – cart – wheel – steering – accident – police – crime –burglar. I explain that in making a conversation one says the first thing that comes into one's head following from what the other person said. So we play the game again using phrases instead of words, for example: Have you had your holiday? I'm going to France in September – Paris is a lovely town – I've never been there – neither have I – I'd like to go but can't afford it – money goes nowhere these days, etc.

I advise patients when at a party or in a pub to be prepared to stand alone and listen, and while doing so to assess the other people and try to see what sort of a person each one might be – this will take their minds off themselves – then to look around for someone else who is standing or sitting alone and go to join them. This person may perhaps be even shyer, so trying to get him or her into conversation will depend upon the patient, and this should give him courage.

ASSESSING NORMALITY

People who have suffered severely from fear, anxiety and worry often find it difficult to accept that a measure of these is a normal component of living. For instance, a patient who had done well and been discharged some six months previously telephoned to say that she had suffered a panic attack. I invited her to attend the next tutorial, and she told us, 'I was on the top of a bus in the main road when it skidded in the snow; it went up on the pavement, just missed a lady with a pram and went in through the shop window. It was dreadful and I had a panic attack'. Less spectacular examples of this reaction are common, such as 'I worry a lot, I wish I could stop'. 'What about?' 'Well my husband has a bad chest so he's been off work a lot, he thinks he'll lose his job. Then the oldest boy is in trouble with the police again and I think he'll go to jail. But the worst thing is the way the girl goes on, I think she'll get pregnant for sure'. Explaining these fears is obviously just a matter of pointing out that life's like that and the patient has similar worries to everyone else. But that as I have stated above, if she faces up to the worst that can happen in any set of circumstances, and resolves that if it should happen she will endure it as best she can, she will find that her worrying will be reduced to reasonable proportions.

7

Errors in the Training for Life

Variations in patterns of training are, of course, infinite. So are individual reactions to any pattern, as is shown by siblings who have received similar treatment in childhood, but have responded differently. I have not, therefore, attempted to exhaust the possibilities but have described some examples to show the lines along which I think when taking a history from a patient.

If the three links in the chain of evidence – symptoms, when and where they occur, the precipitating factor of the illness, and the early training for life – are reviewed in this order (chronologically in reverse), a logical deduction is not usually difficult to make. Having thus deduced the cause(s) of the current symptoms I suggest my explanation to the patient diffidently. I then leave him to think about it at home until next I see him.

In explaining the training error I indulge in fantasy saying, 'It is as if someone taught you to drive on the wrong side of the road on an old airfield, and then sent you alone onto the public road. You would have accident after accident because of your training error, and you would always believe that the other person was wrong. If fact right or wrong do not come into it; you and the other person would just be responding to different training'.

THE SCAPEGOAT

The scapegoat usually has one dominant, violent-tempered parent and one subservient parent. (I have written on the scapegoat in some detail not because it is more common or more important than other patterns of mistraining in childhood, but because it presents enough facets to make it a readily usable model as to how the therapist should think round the whole problem which a patient presents, in an attempt to identify those errors in his training that are causing his symptoms.) A family under pressure of blame and anger from one dominant parent seeks a scapegoat on whom, by common consent, to lay the blame and abreact the aggressions which, initiated at the top of the hierarchy, are generated in all of them. A markedly dominant, irritable parent with a violent temper lays blame unreasonably when irritability arises so though the other parent and the children may strive to be 'good' it is impossible to be good enough to avoid explosions of temper directed at any one of them. Perhaps the seed of the scapegoat pattern is sown when one child, out of his own fear, lies his way out of trouble at the expense of another and gets away with it. As the pattern develops it is as if the subservient parent and the children offer one of their number as a sacrifice to this god of wrath under whose sway they have to live.

By thus directing onto one member of the family the great majority of the anger they generate, the other members of the family can form better relationships with each other than they could if anger were indiscriminately directed. But in order to alleviate their guilt feelings they must establish by mutual consent that the chosen scapegoat is in need of correction and so will benefit by punishment, bullying, or nagging.

In my experience the choice of scapegoat falls most often on a girl and usually on a younger child; but the child who is different from the others, the odd man out, is an obvious choice. So is the child who arouses jealousy in more than one sibling, as is common when a new baby withdraws some of a mother's attention from children aged, say, three to six who have hitherto enjoyed it all. If this baby chances to be of the sex undesired by the parents, or grows to be a physical or temperamental misfit in the family, he or she is an obvious choice for the scapegoat role, while a younger sibling may escape this misfortune. The only child of either sex very occasionally acts as scapegoat for the subservient parent.

Having established the tradition that the scapegoat is substandard in personality and behaviour, the rest of the family must thereafter not admit that the child has done anything right. When he does so, as inevitably he must, his action must be damned with faint praise, made to appear ludicrous or compared unfavourably with the achievement of another. Perhaps he has been accepted for the football team; but his brother is in the cricket team which is considered superior. He must never be allowed to shine or to compete successfully with his siblings in the eyes of the family because this would only arouse guilt. He has to remain the family failure.

The training of the scapegoat thus includes a great deal of criticism; as a result he may learn to be critical in an attempt at self-defence, and this intolerance may cause him to bring down trouble on himself throughout life. It is as if he were an enemy agent in that everyone is against him, so he may respond to this by looking for trouble in all his relationships and therefore finding it. He has been trained to regard himself as substandard, 'difficult' and peculiar; but his sense of justice is likely to cause him to doubt this assessment so he may go into early adult life boldly determined to prove his family wrong. But as his training in forming relationships has been so outstandingly bad, this is likely to cause him failures in this field. He may fall out with his superiors at work and his spouse at home. His family will react by saying that these were only to be expected and the patient, in his own mind, is likely to agree with them and see himself as defeated. It is then that symptoms of neurosis are likely to bring him to psychotherapy.

Betty was seventeen, the fourth of five siblings and the youngest girl, when she was admitted to my care following an overdose. Her father wrote to say that she was a very bad girl, he hoped we would beat her, and he would no longer allow her in his house. That Betty was a scapegoat came out clearly in the history; I explained this to her, and added that now she was gone it was probable that another child would take her place. Six weeks later she told me that her younger brother Billy, aged sixteen was running away to sea, and that it was obvious that this brother had been chosen as the next scapegoat, as she had thought. Within a year no two members of the family were living under the same roof; no semblance of family unity could be maintained in the absence of a child reared to accept the role of scapegoat. Betty did very well, and when I last heard of her she was happily married with children of her own.

It is interesting to note that Billy opted out of the scapegoat role after only six weeks, whereas Betty despaired of herself and took an overdose. This is to be expected because Betty, having been the scapegoat from infancy, at least half-believed that she deserved all this punishment whereas her brother, coming to it at sixteen, believed no such thing. This, then, is the first training error which the scapegoat must correct; he feels that everything which goes wrong is his fault and that he cannot hope to do right.

It is also of note that a family with a scapegoat, while anxious to tell anyone who will listen what a bad child he/she is, will not part with the scapegoat. Friends or acquaintances of the family may offer to take the scapegoat child off their hands, but this offer will be refused on high-minded ethical grounds. It is only when family guilt is evident, as in Betty's case, that a face-saving rejection of the child will be made and another chosen to take the scapegoat role. The scapegoat is very valuable to the family so if he leaves, when he is of an age to do so, attempts, often sentimental, may be made to bring him back. He would be wise to ignore these because if he returns to the bosom of the family his role will again be that of scapegoat.

The scapegoat tends to respond to family demands because he still feels, as he has been taught to feel, that he is essentially bad, but that the family at least will tolerate him whereas he cannot expect acceptance from the general public. His advisers should guard against the error of encouraging him to return to this shaming and humiliating family tolerance, which is the best he is likely to receive. Instead, he would do well to make his own way as a member of the human race, which he is probably amply capable of doing, and only needs to make the attempt while ignoring his feelings to the contrary. His education for lifemanship has been so poor that undoubtedly he will have difficulties in forming relationships; but his courage, once aroused in this direction, will serve to carry him over them. He needs to recognize that he has been handicapped by his education, and will then be able to extend tolerance for his mistakes instead of condemning himself as he has been taught to do. He needs to accept that, under his circumstances, life is bound to be difficult – and then accept the challenge.

As a result of having suffered very considerable injustice the scape-goat may be obsessed with concepts of rights and despise expediency, presumably because he has been at the receiving end of this in the family too often and too much to his disadvantage. In this too he may be making life difficult for himself.

INADEQUACY

A child subjected to the spectacle of violence, ranging from parental–verbal to international high-explosive, seems to be most impressed by his inadequacy to cope with the situation, so he may grow up with a conviction that life is too much for him, thus attracting the label of 'inadequate personality'. He also gives in to other people because he 'doesn't like unpleasantness'. His situation is that of a toothless member of a dog pack. If he can be persuaded that he is in fact no less competent to cope with life than the rest of us he will, apprehensively at first, have a go at something. He protests that he cannot because he has no confidence, so the therapist must explain that confidence only comes with experience, no-one but a fool is confident the first time he sits behind the wheel of a car.

Amnesia for most of the parental rows is common; a patient may remember accompanying his mother to the casualty department on several occasions before he started school, but be unable to remember hearing the fights which led to these episodes. Alternatively, he may be able to describe graphically himself and siblings shivering in their night clothes at the top steps of the stairs while listening in terror to the uproar rising to crescendo below them.

In teaching a patient to stand up for himself I start by teaching him to stand up to me. I say, 'Supposing I said to you, "How dare you come in here in grey trousers and a blue shirt", what would you say to me?' If *he* doesn't know the answer the class does: 'Mind you own business!' We go on to discuss what he might say to people who put on him.

REJECTION

The scapegoat is a rejected child, but many children who are not scape-goats are rejected though the effect of rejection is less if it is shared with siblings.

Rejection, especially of the very young child who is not yet old enough to serve as a scapegoat, strikes terror of death. This is reason-able, as small children are primitive creatures and in nature the rejected young starve. Even today the rejected child is less well cared for and, therefore, more likely to die than the loved child. Napoleon Bonaparte was a bloodthirsty monster who cared not at all for his soldiers' sufferings; but he was the first to put ambulances into the battlefield because he knew that his troops' awareness that they stood a chance of help if wounded would make them fight better. The rejected child goes into the battle of life with no ambulance, so he is often over-cautious with himself, which arouses the contempt of his peers from whom he learns again that he is a substandard human being.

In teaching the rejected patient the therapist is very dependent on his past history, as frequent references to his early training and the inevitable effects they had on him will be needed to persuade him that he is neither substandard nor a coward. He must be persuaded to ignore his terrors while he does what he fears, and to accept the prospect of death as part of life.

PARENTAL PRIDE

Here the patient usually has at least one parent with a marked sense of inferiority for which he compensates. As a result he may be very successful in some activity, but to have a child who is not a success is intolerable to him. Too much is expected of this child who may be very successful, perhaps rarely lower than third in his class, but only top of the class will satisfy the parent so this highly successful child feels a failure. he is intensely competitive in everything he does in adult life and suffers anxiety if he is not succeeding immoderately. He is liable to duck out of situations in which he feels he may fail, such as examinations or interviews, thus causing certain failure. When he understands why he reacts in these ways, that failure is an inevitable part of life and no worse for him than for those he has beaten in the past, he can also learn to accept failure and to do things for the pleasure he gets out of doing rather than for the triumphant end result. This, though always pleasant, is not as important to any of us as the bread and butter of job satisfaction.

THE 'ONLY' CHILD

He is often not actually the only child of his parents, but he may be the oldest or youngest by around five years or more; he is then the only small child in the household during his first five years. He may be the one of a number of siblings lent to a lonely grandmother or aunt; or be the only child of his or her sex, singled out for special treatment on this account; or just be the favourite child of both parents or of the dominant parent; or be the child chosen as mother's companion when father dies or leaves the family.

The problems listed below are not peculiar to 'only' children, but I have found it useful to go through them with each 'only' child referred to me, so I have assembled them under this heading.

Problems of the 'only' child

(1) *Spoiling*. By this is meant not necessarily too many material benefits, but more getting too much of one's own way. This training may lead to difficulty in enduring the minor hardships of life which come to us all. For example, he might receive an electricity or telephone account which he is unable to pay, and feel that bitter injustice has been done to him when the supply is cut off – this sort of thing should not be allowed to happen to him.

(2) *Attention*. The child is constantly under a searchlight of observation and comment because there are no other children to divert parental attention, so self-consciousness is likely to result. More is being expected than he can provide, so feelings of inadequacy may be imprinted.

(3) *Too much is done for him*. It is far easier to do something oneself than to teach someone else to do it, and to watch a small child fumbling with shoelaces or buttons takes patience, so the only child may not be allowed to learn such simple skills at the normal age. If there were an older child to be got ready to school, and/or a younger one needing a nappy change, the mother would be thankful to see him start to fumble for himself. Training in dependency may result and inferiority feelings when he compares his abilities with those of children of his age.

(4) *Loneliness*. This only occurs in crowded areas in the presence of invalidism or parental possessivenss, but it often occurs amongst the better housed and country dwellers. The child may fail to learn to mix, and dislike of school may follow.

(5) *Inferiority/inadequacy*. All children are inferior and inadequate compared with adults. If there is at least one other child with whom to share this state the child accepts it as normal, which it is; but if there is no other child the habit of seeing himself as inferior may become fixed. Perhaps this is more likely to occur in a household containing a number of older people, including siblings of school age at the time of the subject's birth; he is then so far outdistanced that it may seem to him that he will never catch up.

(6) *Subjection to others*. This may be marked in a child reared in a household containing a number of adults and children much older than himself if domination is the usual pattern of family behaviour.

(7) *Mistrust of the object of his affections*. This may occur in the 'only' child who is also the oldest in the family because, at five years old or a little more, he is intensely aware of parental betrayal when the first

sibling is born. At that age his attachment to his parents is still undivided; to find their attachment to *him* divided is a shattering experience.

(8) *Parental quarrelling.* This is liable to affect the 'only' child more than if he is one of several siblings.

(9) *Standing up for one's self.* This is a lesson first learned on the nursery floor – Sue snatches Tom's bunny and pulls its ear off, so Tom hits Sue. The 'only' child may miss out on this, and find it difficult to learn in later life.

Obviously it would be a very unlucky child that suffered *all* these training errors; those he does suffer depend on circumstances.

THE MISFIT

Let us call him or her Jo. The misfit doesn't fit his family; there is nothing much wrong with the child, he would fit another family, nor is there much wrong with the family, another child would fit in it; indeed the fact that other children do fit in it is one of Jo's worries about himself. It's just that Jo is different from the others, he may be more or less intelligent more or less practical, more or less artistic. The same phenomenon occurs in litters of puppies; it is not uncommon to have a level litter, temperament-wise, with an odd one – this may be the genius or the dunce, the bully or the bullied.

Because Jo is different he's awkward, a square peg in a round hole; naturally the family tries to rub off his corners, but he keeps growing new ones, and they never know what he'll be up to next. It's not that what he does is always or especially mischievous, but to the family it is unexpected because it does not conform to what they do. So Jo grows up in an atmosphere of disapproval which, most of the time, may be gently expressed by the parents; but sibling rivalry for parental approval is likely to cause attention to be drawn to Jo's 'faults' more often than is good for him. He can do nothing right, so he comes to believe himself to be 'bad', though he strives to alter this which leads to being made use of by the family. Thus he is tolerated, belittled and despised, and any time there is a nasty job to do he gets it, and does it.

At play, at school and, ultimately, at work Jo finds relationships with other people much more rewarding than are those with his family. For others he *can* do right, they don't disapprove of him, or make him feel he is bad. So Jo starts to drift away from the family a little which the latter doesn't like; he's not there to be made use of when he *should* be, so the family protests. At this point Jo starts to pay back what he owes, he tells them their faults and how horrible they have been to him. Of course, parents and siblings are deeply hurt, they are united in their conviction that they are good and Jo is bad, they have tolerated him with exemplary fortitude for all these years and he is now biting the hand that fed him! They wail about Jo to anyone who will listen, and as a result the area of disapproval around Jo widens to include other relatives and friends, so Jo drifts further away.

Sooner or later a do-gooder related to or associated with the family tells Jo, more in sorrow than in anger, how unkind he is to his loving family and how ungrateful for all the blessings that the family has showered upon him. Attempting to defend himself against this attack Jo quotes episodes from his own past which do not show the family in a very good light. He is then condemned for nursing grievances and being disloyal, which makes him realize that, in the context of loyalty and grievance, what is sauce for the goose is evidently not sauce for the gosling.

He is likely to leave this interview filled with a burning sense of injustice, so if he gets drunk, hits a policeman, steals a car and ends up in jail, no wonder. Or if she gets drunk, goes on the streets and gets pregnant it is only what one might expect. The family says to Jo, self-righteously of course, 'We told you so'.

The court, perhaps, refers Jo for a psychiatric opinion, so he arrives in my office sulky, shamefaced, expecting another reproval. I say, 'Tell me the story, perhaps I can help'. Stumbling at first, and later warming to the task, helped by occasional questions, he tells his tale. When the picture has become clear I suggest, hesitantly, that he might care to consider the notion, 'Look out for yourself, because if you don't nobody else will'.

While discussing this new idea Jo may point out that one should consider other people first. I suggest that if one gets one's feet firmly planted one might be more competent to consider others, adding that there's no sense in jumping off a pier to help a drowning man if one hasn't first learned to swim. Before parting I may or may not remark that getting drunk, hitting policemen and stealing cars (or going on the streets and getting pregnant) are perhaps not the best ways to look out for oneself, but Jo will already be thinking that.

When we part I ask whether he would like to see me again; if I have struck the right notes the answer will be 'Yes', and I can make the appropriate recommendation to the court.

I should remind my readers at this point that I am writing about neurotics, not psychopaths. Had Jo hit a policeman or stolen a car when unprovoked and sober my reactions might be very different.

THE OVERPROTECTED CHILD OF
THE CLOSE-KNIT FAMILY

Probably the parents of such a family fear any form of strife, so normal childish quarrels and tantrums are treated 'more in sorrow than in anger', which is devastating. The christianity of 'Gentle Jesus meek and mild', rather than that of he who ejected crooked dealers with a whip, is likely to be taught in such a home. No word is spoken in anger and no unkind word about anyone is permitted. The family climate is stiflingly close rather than cosy.

Educating a child of such a family lacks realism with regard to human nature, independence and self-defence, which leaves the subject ill-equipped to cope with ordinary people. Tears are his only defence against any form of aggression, and neurotic anxiety follows any prolonged or repeated experience of aggression or even absence of loving support.

Persuading such a patient that life will never be a bed of thornless roses is usually difficult but not impossible. Being made of common clay the patient responds to aggression with aggression of a kind not recognized by him as such – withdrawing, weeping, passive resistance and sulking are likely patterns of behaviour. When awareness dawns these patterns are converted into more overt aggression which is both beneficial to the patient and more tolerable to his associates. When he has thus learned to stand up for himself openly, and accepted the necessity to do so, he is capable of coping with ordinary life.

Twins

A similar pattern is liable to occur in the case of twins, in whom reliance on each other may be such that they contrive to isolate themselves from their normal share of 'slings and arrows' in the school playground. There may be such interdependence that if one is better than the other in work or sport, any advancement may be rejected so the pair can remain together; for instance, one or both may deliberately spoil examination papers. The pattern may continue at work so that separation comes only with marriage. Of course, the spouse is likely to be a less wholehearted emotional supporter than was the twin, so it is then the subject developes anxiety symptoms and, hopefully, starts re-education.

THE PATIENT'S PARENTS

In teaching patients about their childhoods I am careful to absolve their parents of blame. I also avoid suggesting that they owe any family loyalty or that their families are likely to be of any emotional help in their problems. I advise them not to discuss what they are learning from me with their parents or other relations.

Many people, who have been much more fortunate in their early family relationships than most of my patients, and who treat or aspire to treat neurotics, feel that family unity is of obvious benefit especially to those in trouble. 'Your best friends will always be your parents,' they say. In treating neurotics, however, such an attitude is positively damaging. The patient's best hope of recovery is to escape, at least temporarily, from all family demands and traditions. The therapist's first duty is to act in the best interests of the patient's recovery.

Pity for parents who, by the time the patient comes for treatment, may be poor old folks who insist, probably truthfully, that they are fond of him, is no excuse for delaying the patient's recovery. When he has won his fight he can make his own emotional and ethical decisions and should be left to do so.

If a patient's progress is delayed by misplaced loyalty to parents, I point out that his first duty is to make the most of himself as an efficient human being; only then will he be better placed to help his parents if help is needed, but that all our most pressing debts are to *future* generations.

If relatives ask to see me I do so only with the patient's consent, and the reassurance that I will not divulge anything he has told me. I am very careful to say nothing to them which, in garbled version, may be fed back to the patient prefaced by 'Doctor says. . .'. I prefer not to see relatives of neurotics at all, because I want there to be no possibility of error as to whose side I am on. In this I make an exception in favour of spouses, but I prefer to see the couple together.

8

Relationships

Problems in relationships are universal in neurosis, and are the immediate causes of the fears. It is impossible to offer a comprehensive account of the method here, but an attempt will be made in this chapter

In a tutorial a patient brings up a problem in his relationship with another person who may be a friend, relation or fellow worker, either peer or superior. The therapist asks 'Why did X say or do that?', eliciting generally a superficial answer which probably infers the assumption that X was right. Discussion with the therapist, sometimes helped by the other patients, continues until some understanding of X's possible motives and/or neurotic reactions is reached. Or the appropriate question from the therapist to the patient may be, 'Why did you react as you did?' The answer is less superficial but probably infers that the patient was wrong. Discussion is directed towards self-understanding and self-respect, and suggestions as to what that patient might, with advantage, have said or done may be made by both therapist or patients. There is rarely a need for the therapist to direct the patient's thoughts towards self-blame, he does that all too readily for himself; or if he is guilty and cannot face it, he may find himself more able to do so because the therapist has inferred that no guilt exists. If he verbalizes guilt which the therapist sees as justified, it must be explained that the therapist has either done the same sort of thing, or probably would have given the patient's circumstances, which are then recapitulated starting from childhood if appropriate.

In such conversations, and similar ones between the therapist and other patients, the patient is absorbing the idea that he is not necessarily always wrong nor are other people always right. As a result he is learning to assess other people, to see himself as less of an oddity, and thus to move in the direction of normal assertion in relationships. As he advances, there may be excess assertion, to the point of verbal aggression. He is advised to let it look after itself, and is told that when he has advanced further into self-assurance his pity will moderate his aggression. The difference between inhibition of aggression through fear, and moderation of aggression through pity, or for reasons of expediency, is explained.

THE PATIENT WHO IS ALWAYS PUT UPON

A patient who is anxious about a relationship problem often wants to tell a very long and involved story. I have found it unwise to let this flow uninterrupted, because by the time we have finally reached the end, we have missed a number of discussion points and, even if I have made notes of these, it is difficult for the patient to remember precisely what he said. So I interrupt, we discuss a point, and the patient continues. I may interrupt several times, always using the same technique to get the patient to think more deeply about motives and ethics. The following interchange gives some idea of the technique used.

Patient . . . so Mother cried and said she had done without a drink of tea for three days because I hadn't brought her any; but I *couldn't* get down with two children in bed with 'flu and the 'bus strike, and one of them really bad, and Mrs Brown would have got her tea if she'd said so. . . .
Therapist Just stop there a moment. Why did your mother say that about the tea?
Patient She thought I should have got it.
Therapist Yes, but why did she *say* it? Why did she rub it in? Do *you* always remind other people of things they haven't done when you know they've had troubles themselves, especially when you have, or could have, got over the difficulty?
Patient No . . . no, I don't; but Mother's always like that.
Therapist Yes, always has been since you can remember! . . . Tell me, why did she do without tea when Mrs Brown would have got it?
Patient I don't know; but she's like that.
Therapist Yes, but think . . . why did she do without tea?

The patient shakes her head helplessly, being afraid to answer in what she feels to be a treasonable way.

Therapist   Can anyone tell her?
Second patient   She did it to make you sorry, to make you ashamed, to punish you for not going to see her for three days . . . three days! Can't she get out to the shops?
Patient   Yes but she doesn't like to when it's cold.
Second patient   Neither do I!
Therapist   Why did she want to make you sorry and ashamed?
Patient   She thinks mothers should come first.
Therapist   Would you expect it of your children?
Patient (emphatically)   I hope I never do.
Therapist   What might you have said to her?
Patient   Well I told her I couldn't help it because. . . .
Therapist   Yes; but what *might* you have said?

The patient doesn't answer so I ask the class

Third patient   She might have told her she was a wicked, selfish, unkind old woman!

A group discussion on what people owe to parents follows, in the course of which I state my opinion, which is fallible but supported by the scriptures, to the effect that we owe it to parents to see that their physical needs are supplied when they can no longer supply these for themselves, but we do not necessarily have to do this personally. I add that if parents have made friends of their children it is likely that the latter will do much more than this for their own pleasure and in the name of friendship; but that, with the one exception mentioned, all our debts are to the future, to the rising generation, to our children if we have any, or to society if we have none.

I usually wind up the discussion by saying to the patient, 'You take the old girl a bit too seriously don't you? She's just a naughty old woman who likes her own way, isn't she? She knows you are soft, and she's only got to be sorry for herself to get you running around her. You might try laughing at her a little. Next time you see her say, with a bright smile, "Had any tea?" Let her see that she's not going to get you worried as easily as all that.'

In tutorials on problems of relationships or self-management patients are asked to state the problem as simply and briefly as they can, and then advised to restate the problem to themselves frequently and consider solutions. In this way they should try to be concise and productive rather than allow themselves to burble on pointlessly about their grievances, however real these may be.

THE PATIENT WHO IS BUYING LOVE

The most common cause of problems of interpersonal relationships is, of course, the patients' fear of losing love through assertion. As a result they forfeit respect and cause irritation. I tell them two stories.

1. 'If you had a dog without any teeth, and you took him for a walk, he would cringe at your heel with his tail between his legs looking anxiously sideways at every other dog, which would encourage the other dogs to go for him. But if you put his teeth back in his head and took him out he'd run along waving his tail with his tongue hanging out happily; he wouldn't start a fight, but because he knew that if necessary he could defend himself he wouldn't be worried.'

2. 'Many years ago in this country the Danes came in their ships. They robbed, burnt, raped, murdered and carried home slaves. The government agreed to pay them a large tax called Danegeld so that they would stay away. The Danes collected the tax, but still returned to rob, burn, rape and murder just the same.'

I ask 'What do you want love for?' The usual answer is that it makes the patient feel safe. I point out that this feeling is a lie and that the Saxons paid the Danegeld to feel safe. I say that small children need love to feel safe, because they feel that if they aren't loved they will be abandoned to starve, and that, even today, they are right, the unloved child is at greater risk than the loved child; but that when we are grown-up we don't *need* love, though we always like to have it. If we didn't get enough love when we were little we developed the habit of trying to buy it, which the patient is still doing; but this never pays because people, including our children, despise us for behaving childishly. I advise the patient to start looking for respect rather than love – the latter will come naturally in the presence of respect.

The patient then says that getting respect means having rows and he hates rows. I point out that having rows takes courage, that the first time he stands up for himself he will be terrified, but that this will become easier with practice. He says he never can think of the right things to say; I reply that it doesn't matter much what he says, it's *how* he says it, it's the fact that he's not giving in.

Dependence on love

The mass media thrives on romance; insecure people crave love and derive some satisfaction from contemplating others receiving it. As a result there is widespread belief that love is as necessary to the survival of the adult as, say, air or water. So it comes as a shock to most patients when I tell them that adults don't need love any more than they need ice cream or alcohol.

Dependence on love leads to the demand for love which, if excessive, kills it, thus destroying the total relationship in many cases. The belief that love is essential justifies the manipulation of others; thus parents may keep their growing or grown-up children in an inferior and dependent position so that the children continue to need and love them.

THE PATIENT WHO NEEDS EMOTIONAL SUPPORT

The following conversation gives an idea how I deal with this kind of patient.

Patient Do you know, when I was in bed with a bad cold my sister wouldn't even come and make me a cup of tea!
Therapist Couldn't you make one yourself?
Patient Yes, of course I did; but I was upset.

We talked around this until she could see for herself that what she wanted was to know that her sister cared; she was looking for a prop.

Therapist What do you want support for?
Patient Because it makes me feel better.
Therapist What way better?
Patient Safer I suppose.
Therapist What way safer?
Patient (after thought) What would happen if I was too ill to get to the kitchen?

Therapist What does happen to people who are too ill to look after themselves and have no-one to look after them?

We reach the conclusion that they go to hospital. So we get back to her feeling that she needs someone to lean on.

Therapist Now just think, do you really need this support? It won't stop you getting pneumonia, it won't stop the house burning down; but it will leave you with a debt to your sister, whereas if you look after yourself you owe nothing. Might it not be better to stand on your own feet?

Patient But surely we all depend on someone?

Therapist On whom do we all depend? We all depend on the public services and on many of our neighbours who also depend on us. We rely on the milkman to bring the milk, on the gas company, the dustbin man, the baker, the butcher and a lot more; but we pay for these services so it leaves us free of moral debts. Thus we are independent adults, not little children being dependent on other people whom we then have to obey. [We talk round that a bit.] Apart from these services for which you pay what you want of other people?

The answers are usually help in an emergency such as the house burning down, common courtesy and companionship.

THE PATIENT WHO BULLIES

This patient complains that he bullies his spouse and children, although he regrets doing so. He may even attempt to bully his psychotherapist. I point out that anyone who feels inferior also feels that anyone who accepts him must be inferior because superior people would reject him. So he feels safe in bullying those who accept him and, in doing so, only treats them as *he* expects to be treated. The climate of hatred in which the child was reared teaches him two things: first to hate, and second that aggressive behaviour in the home is normal. So he acts out his hatred on those who accept him and thus kills the love he craves. He is afraid to act out his hatred on those whom he feels to be superiors, and these probably include his parents.

The man or woman who, as a child, has been bullied, chided and derided to excess finds it difficult to love even his or her own child. It is by inspiring in him pity and mercy *for the child that he was*, as opposed to the learned self-condemnation which, though unacknowledged, has become habitual, that kindness can overcome harshness, first to himself and then to others. So sometimes the chain of hatred which passes from generation to generation and leads to physically or mentally battered children, wives and husbands can be broken.

As long as people hate themselves they will hate others, but is not usually beyond their capacities to learn the more pleasant prospect of loving themselves.

It is important to note that the neurotic's self-condemnation or hatred is unacknowledged, in fact there is often compensation so the façade presented may even be 'holier than thou'. And as self-hatred, being of lifelong duration, does not strike the patient as being abnormal, he is unlikely to be consciously aware of it at least until well into the treatment. To the discerning, however, its presence is apparent, through self-consciousness, apology and sometimes bombast.

THE PATIENT WHO IS MORALLY DEFICIENT

I must remind readers that in this book I am writing about *neurotics*, not *psychopaths*. A hallmark of the psychopath is that he or she loves and pities himself all too well, having a remarkable talent for inspiring pity in others. Reading reports on children battered to death while under social service supervision, I have sometimes been struck by the ease with which the psychopathic parent has conned the social worker. The psychopath carries conviction because he himself believes that he cannot be wrong – other people are *always* wrong! He deserves a certain amount of pity for being psychopathic, but the pity which he so easily inspires may be disastrous to others.

Case history

Description of the thought processes of one psychopath may perhaps be appropriate for comparison with that of neurotics. Many years ago I treated a psychopath, a large, strong young man, married with two young children. He was often unfaithful, explaining that he couldn't help this, he just loved 'loving', which he thought perfectly all right; but he also 'loved' his wife, so when she was concerned he was very jealous. His own nocturnal adventures of course gave her opportunity to repay him in kind so, though he had no reason to think her unfaithful, he punished her physically to keep her on the 'straight and narrow'. He thought this harmless because he didn't actually break her bones. His wife left him and started divorce proceedings, initially with an injunction to stop him coming to her house and hitting her. He explained that he did this because, naturally, he needed his wife's love and support and was angry with her for leaving him. When he had broken the injunction several times the police intervened, which he thought very wrong of them – the police should not intervene in domestic quarrels. In due course he went to jail for breaking the injunction; this he well knew was the probable outcome, but he found it cruelly wrong on the part of his wife, and asked her how she could be so wicked as to torture him in this way.

The case history above well illustrates the inability to assess cause and effect, the impulsiveness and the firm belief that everything that goes wrong is the fault of someone else. To oversimplify: the neurotic thinks he is *wrong* when he isn't, but the psychopath thinks he is *right* when he isn't; the neurotic blames himself unduly, where the psychopath blames others and/or circumstances, anyone *but* himself; the neurotic misses opportunities through hesitancy, while the psychopath acts immediately on the impulse of the moment. When considering psychopathy one can only say, 'There, but for the grace of God go I', and then strive to curtail the damage they do to others.

THE PATIENT WHO NAGS

She (sometimes he) compensates for her sense of inferiority, and finds outlets for the irritation resulting from inferiority feelings by putting people to rights. She learned that this behaviour was adult-superior by being at the receiving end of it herself, and probably first practised it on younger siblings; for this she may have received commendation and prefect status in the home because such behaviour in an older child saves mother some trouble. If she suffered pangs of jealousy over a younger sibling she may have abused this status without receiving parental censure. Thus she is convinced that nagging is right, so if someone says to her, 'For God's sake stop it!' she replies with complete sincerity, 'But I'm only trying to help!' Take, for example, the following conversation.

Therapist Do you think you nag your husband?
Patient He says so, but it doesn't seem like that to me.

Therapist What did you last nag him about?
Patient He left the door open, there was a draught.
Therapist Did you have a bit of a row?
Patient I am afraid we did.
Therapist Might it be less trouble to shut the door yourself?
Patient But it's *wrong* to leave doors open!
Therapist (with a grin and a wink):   A lot of things are wrong, but life isn't long enough to put them all right. Rows are nasty, God won't punish you for your husband's sins, you need to look out for yourself a bit more. (And, having given that time to sink in) Tell me, did they nag you a lot when you were a child?
Patient Only for my own good.
Therapist If it's now causing rows was it all that good, or did it just teach you the habit of finding fault?

Provided that the inferiority feelings are being treated successfully and concurrently the seed thus sown stands a chance of germinating.

The therapist acts on the assumption that the customer is always right, so he presents matters from that angle. Quoting from *Punch*:

Lady choosing shoes   I think one of my feet is bigger than the other.
Shop assistant Oh no, Madam, smaller if anything.

MARITAL RELATIONSHIPS

It is common for two neurotics to marry each other. The person who is emotionally insecure feels for the fellow sufferer and enjoys a sense of equality with a person whose inferiority feelings he is subconsciously aware of, hence the initial bond.

But emotional insecurity demands support which the fellow sufferer is more likely to demand than to give, while the sense of mutual equality frees both to address criticisms towards each other which neither would venture to do towards someone who, in their eyes, ranked as superior. And, having no fear of each other, anger aroused by others is likely to be vented on the spouse rather than on one who aroused it. 'The blind lead the blind and thus shall they both fall into the ditch' of marital disharmony.

If disharmony leads to violence it is usually the woman who seeks support from her family doctor who may refer her for psychiatry. Even in the absence of violence it is more often the woman than the man who seeks help, with the added motive of desire for continued financial support if her children are very young. A sense of guilt over the failure of the marriage may be apparent, perhaps exacerbated by frigidity resulting either from rejection or from the couple's failure to develop postnatal sexual techniques. Rejection can, of course, cause impotence.

It is common for married couples to regard mutual criticism as normally acceptable social behaviour. While admitting that this may be so I point out that a critical climate often plays a large part in the breakdown of a marriage, because if competitive it turns the association into one long row, or if onesided the recipient is likely to say, 'I can't do anything right so I may as well get out'. I ask the patient, 'Do you criticize your boss at work?' Of course he answers, 'No, I want to keep my job!' So I ask, 'If you took a friend out and spent the evening discussing his/her faults do you think you might lose that friend?' The answer is 'Probably'. I then point out that losing a spouse is likely to cause far more disturbance than losing a job or a friend because it may include loss of home and/or children, so I advise strong resistance of the urge to criticize the spouse.

Patients sometimes come to the classes to complain at length of their spouse's behaviour. I tell them they have two choices: they can put up with it or they can get out; what they cannot do is alter the spouse. After that point has been grasped, probably as a result of repetition over a period, I modify this statement by explaining that change in the patient, which occurs as a result of treatment, may bring about change in the spouse, which hopefully will be for the better.

If treatment proceeds successfully the change in the patient will be in the direction of increased emotional independence which may be either welcomed or resisted by the spouse. If the spouse is normally emotionally secure the change will be welcomed, but a spouse who is deriving compensation for feelings of inferiority from the patient's dependency and ill-health will resent such a change. Evidence of such resentment is likely to be presented at the classes, so the therapist can then suggest that the patient take every opportunity to pay compliments on everyday matters, such as a well-cooked meal, a proficient handyman job, or an attractive new garment. He or she should take less for granted, say 'thank you' more often, and show more appreciation and affection. Hopefully, this will supply the needed emotional support.

9

Patients and their Comments

PATIENT 1; MARRIED WOMAN, BORN 1946

Diagnosis: Anxiety neurosis.

Attendances: 38 during 8 months, 1975–76. Some individual treatment while travelling home in therapist's car. History: taken when patient was referred in June 1975, at age 29.

Complained of: Frightened of teaching, of supervision, of telephoning, of responsibility, of children.

History of previous complaints: Started at age 5 years, frightened to go to school, and has been frightened of this and that ever since, mainly related to what people think. Started two years' psychotherapy at the Tavistock Clinic, at age 23. In the patient's view no progress, perhaps in reverse. May Day Hospital, Croydon 1973, Moorhaven Hospital 1973, E.C.T. × 10 temporary improvement.

Family history: Father treated for depression.

Background: Own house, husband in part-time employment.

Childhood: Parents didn't quarrel, though there was tension. Close to father, not to mother; patient 29 years, brother 28 years, sister 25 years, sister 21 years. Very close to brother. Father strict – very puritanical – afraid to displease him. He set very high standards. Also afraid to get ideas above her station.

113

School: From 3 ½ years. Very nervous at school, didn't like it, afraid of the other children. Became happy in the 5th form. Good at swimming, hated other games. One friend throughout school, and made a few more but not many. Prefect and vice-captain. Nine O levels, three A levels. Degree in Arts, General Honours, Diploma of Education.

Work: Started age 22 years. Teaching for 1 year – gave up because of panic, since then, cash register–secretarial training – commerce, Civil Service for 2 years – very bored. Now a cashier.

Sex: Boy friends from age 16 years – had fun. Married 1972 aged 26 years, sexually unsatisfactory because she is not physically attracted to her husband, but he doesn't love her intellectually which matters a lot to her. Husband is very artistic and unpractical but she is very fond of him. He is generally helpful to her.

Follow-up: November 1978. Writes that she is considering remarriage when her divorce is absolute and, with regard to work, that she is enjoying the challenge which she always dreaded.

Author's precis of patient 1's comments, received in 1977

I was not a happy child though my parents did their best for us. I didn't know why I was unhappy, but knew I was afraid of everybody and of most situations outside my home. When I was 11 I made an attempt to improve matters. By staying at home the problem of fear would be solved, so I feigned fainting on several occasions while out with my parents. I saw the doctor, was referred to a psychiatrist and stayed at home for some long time. My fears were alleviated but I was no happier, and in the end I got bored and asked to go back to school.

At university I made my next attempt to find out what was wrong with me. I was then still miserable and desperate though not so afraid. I saw the doctor in the student health centre who treated me as rather a nuisance, I being one of many students complaining of 'depressions'. He prescribed tranquillisers which I didn't take because I didn't think them the answer.

About a year later I started work teaching and my uneasiness immediately became tremendously exaggerated. My GP sent me to the hospital where Valium and later Librium were prescribed in increasing doses without relief. I found no answers to my misery nor to the questions in my head – 'Why did I not enjoy life? Why was I so nervous of simple situations and people? Why could I not work happily?' Eventually I was referred to the Tavistock Clinic which I was told had a nationwide if not international reputation.

I waited 6 months for an appointment during which I gave up my new job, though I had passed my probationary teaching year very satisfactorily, but could no longer face the tortures I had gone through. I went to work as a sales assistant where I had rest from the external worries so I had only the internal ones. I began to fear that I was incurable though I tried hard to be happy.

At the Tavistock I was offered a course of weekly 1-hour visits which I attended for 2 years. I started with new hope but I did not know what was expected of me and my initial constraint increased very quickly to total silence. I could not talk and was not spoken to by the therapist from whom I received no encouragement and no explanation, I could only express my increasing distress in tears. One day I offered a written copy of my dreams; I was asked why I did so to which I replied that I thought they might help, but they remained unread. We returned to what became an intolerable silence. Eventually I left, I was probably much more distressed than ever before, even the Tavistock couldn't help me, I must be a fraud. I was then 25.

A year later an unfortunate love affair and marriage to a man I did not love drove me to despair. I took to my bed as a cry for help and was admitted to hospital. There I was given five electroconvulsive treatments and about ten different drugs. I saw the doctors who told me I was nervous, lacked confidence and could only help myself. I tried to pull myself together and when I was discharged we left London for Plymouth. There I again took to my bed not caring to do, see or feel anything. I was admitted to hospital for more electroconvulsions and drugs, also lectures and blue movies designed to increase the desire for my husband which had never existed. The demoralizing atmosphere, the rest from the emotional problems of my marriage and, perhaps, the uplifting effect of the treatment led me to seek discharge. I had learned nothing which would dispel my discontent with life.

My husband was very kind and encouraging, his warmth helped me to overcome my bitterness against those who had claimed to try to help me and failed. We moved from Plymouth to Colne in Lancashire. Two years later I decided to try, just once more, to sort out my difficulties and my GP got me an appointment with a psychiatrist at Burnley.

When I was referred for group psychotherapy I had grave doubts
having heard this treatment scathingly discussed. *

Patient's comments verbatim

"It is difficult to recall exactly how my 'cure' began to evolve. I
attended group therapy for 2 hours a week and continued to attend
for 8 months. Gradually I began to understand why I had been
miserable for 29 years. Over the weeks it was pointed out to me by
the therapist that I had never been free to be myself and that this was
an unwarranted imposition on the part of my elders. My desire to
please my parents, their friends and my teachers rendered me
incapable of making independent decisions. The expectations of
these elders coincided so frequently to negate my own conflicting
desires as to render my 'self' worthless. I tried to have no self as my
'self' did not fit what was expected of me and in the end I fairly succeeded. But how could I have known that that was why I was
unhappy? All my failures combined to strengthen my feelings of
worthlessness, so that were I even to think I wanted something other
than what I was told I *should* want, that thought was worthless in
itself. A vicious circle indeed.

Now for the first time it was pointed out to me that I doubted the
value of all my actions not because they were poor in themselves but
because I still thought them not good enough to please those around
me. I had taken upon myself the standards set by my parents and
teachers as the criterion by which to judge my every move and
thought. And as, when a child, I had never seemed to be able to do
well enough to please these people so, as an adult, I thought that any
standard I could reach was not high enough. I was building in to my
whole way of life a failure factor, and how could anyone living
according to this self-contradictory code fail to be miserable? It was
now pointed out to me that standards are arbitrary and can be
moved up and down and that it makes little sense to live according to
a hard and fast set of rules based on something so unreal. No wonder
I was neurotic! But why should my parents have insisted upon this
method of upbringing? They saw, as I had seen, that without
motivation to action people became cabbages and depressed beings

*The precis was made because the original was too long for publication. It was made
mostly by putting together questions from the patient's script; this has been scrupulously
done in her description of Burnley therapists' work. A copy of the original is retained in
the records.

with no feelings of self-respect. It seemed to them that the setting of standards which could continually be raised would provide the motivation for action towards a good level of achievement. This they had accordingly adopted as their own code of thought and behaviour and also passed on to their children as one they thought most likely to make them happy. They also benefited from the side-effect this produced of their children's 'good' behaviour, so the continuation of this method of training was reinforced.

What they had not understood, although they too were significantly unhappy following this course, was the built-in unhappiness factor which it entailed – the unattainable standard factor. Since they were afraid that without this factor they would lose all motivation to valuable action they, and I in my turn, were much too afraid to drop these standards. And now, once again for the first time, since all the people I had hitherto met were caught in the same trap or did not see that they were caught in it, I was shown what should have been obvious before if I had taken a look, for example, at animal behaviour; that any normal human being who is not building in his own unhappiness factor in the shape of standards set by society has a natural motivation to do things well. Doing things well does not require a standard of achievement to be set. Animals do things well. They do not set themselves standards. Healthy animals are also naturally active and very uncommonly fail to be accepted by others of their kind. And so it is with human beings. In fact, the setting of standards actually inhibits motivation, since the continued frustration of achievement will eventually wear down the will to act, or at least make the natural machinery of motivation, reward and re-motivation work very inefficiently. Standards will eventually create a neurotic even out of the strongest and luckiest of people and animals.

The other way of working things out, which was now presented to me for the first time in my life, is to allow feelings and events to guide the natural development of motivation and desire to act, and I began to dare for the first time to try out this new way of thinking. After all, I could lose nothing, and I had the support of people who were willing to help if I went wrong. So I dared at last to throw away standards and see if things worked well without them. And they did. I began to be happy for the first time. I was free to be me and to discover what I really wanted for the first time. I was 'cured'."

Why had the psychiatrists I had seen before not been able to help? The people at Burnley gave the clue to this by comparison between them and those who went before. Those at Burnley were people of great verbal ability who worked hard to communicate and to make sure that what they said had been understood. They worked on the assumption that neurotics were not basically different from 'normal' people. They disposed of using drugs knowing that this would involve them in a lot of hard work. They were, above all, prepared to show that they did not regard themselves as superior human beings, this argues that they must be pretty convinced of their own value, which convinced their patients that they themselves could be of value to themselves.

They had the answer and they gave it. The surprising thing is that they were the first to see that the answer was so simple. The main reason for this is, I think, that many psychiatrists are not emotionally self-sufficient themselves but depend on the affirmation of their continuing superiority over others to maintain their sense of security.

I was ill because I didn't know that I was capable of emotional self-support and self-stimulus and so was potentially capable of being an autonomous, self-sufficient being. I began to learn this when the therapists not only listened to what I had to say but appeared to learn from it. The frank demonstration by the therapists of weakness balanced by strength as a sufficient basis for self-support was necessary to me before I was convinced that self-sufficiency was a real possibility and not just a theory whose implementation might lead to inevitable disaster, being foreign to the nature of human beings.

I do not think I could have learned this only by attending groups, I think I needed the individual contact with a therapist which I also received.

I believe that the modern insistence, by psychological theorists and those of the 'pop scene', upon the dependence of the adult on love to make him happy, reinforces the lack of confidence in the self which makes it more difficult to accept the philosophy of self-sufficiency.

PATIENT 2, BACHELOR, BORN 1942

Diagnosis: Anxiety neurosis, obsessional features, obsessional personality.

Attendances: 43 during twelve months, 1974–75. University graduate, successful professional man.

The following is a letter dated 3 May 1978.

"By the time I saw you I had been through the hands of a number of other psychiatrists and had consumed a large quantity of 'pills' ranging from amphetamines to tranquillisers. I was suffering from a fairly unpleasant obsessional state which was making my life very difficult, and also was extremely preoccupied about my health. In short I suppose that my neurosis had just about taken over my life. The advice which I had received up to that point was more or less just to carry on with my various medications and everything would be all right, which decidedly it was not.

Looking back it is always difficult to say why but these things just came to a head. I was starting to rely on drink and finally I gave up (ran away from) my job and went back to the bosom of my parents.

That really produced more stress as my family were unable to understand why I had given up a 'bright' future for what appeared to them to be very 'airy fairy' reasons.

It was in those circumstances that I met you and came into contact with your method.

I must admit that initially I was rather sceptical when I heard that your method of treatment consisted merely of group discussion (or so I thought).

Now, two years after finishing treatment with you, I am back at my job and am virtually symptom-free and most important of all I feel able to control these symptoms which I still have.

The lessons which I learnt from your groups will stick with me for life and being at your groups was one of the most worthwhile experiences in my life. One starts by being ashamed of being neurotic and one ends by realizing that it gives one an added perspective of life.

What did I learn from your groups? I think above all I learned for the first time to understand why I had become neurotic which I had never understood before. Before it had always seemed as if my problems were rather like 'flu, just a chance germ which I had caught. I now realize that given the circumstances in which I had been brought up and the aspirations and demands made by my parents it was inevitable that I should have ended up as I did.

I also began to realize that I was not alone and that others, due to little fault of their own, were in exactly the same situation as I was.

Most important of all I learned how to accept the worst that could happen and get on with life and cope. This fairly quickly got rid of my hypochondria – one simply accepts that the worst that can happen is that one can die and one learns not to waste time worrying about it.

You never gave any of us sympathy but you did give us tremendous support.''

PATIENT 3, MARRIED WOMAN, BORN 1930

Diagnosis: Anxiety neurosis.

Attendances: 51 in 1977–78, at age 47. History: taken when patient was referred in July 1977.

Complained of: Slight depression, 'all on edge', restless, panic when she goes out, then feels a fool. Worries about furnishings, carpet spoilt, etc. Can't drop off easily but sleeps till time to get up. No symptoms of endogenous depression.

History of previous complaints: In 1951 was depressed for 2 years following child's death; 1964 hysterectomy followed by depression, symptoms as above, also early waking and cancerophobia. ECT × 8 with improvement. Readmitted six months later with present symptoms only. ECT × 12 without improvement. Symptoms continued 1964–68, treated as outpatient with Triptafen and Valium. Between 1968–71 not attending clinic, at her own wish, no medication but symptoms continued. In 1971 exacerbation of symptoms with choking and inability to swallow, treated by GP with Triptafen which was continued for five years. In 1976 arthritis in her back with exacerbation of symptoms. Triptafen discontinued by GP who substituted for it other antidepressants and tranquillisers, but, in the patient's opinion, nothing would replace Triptafen.

Family history: Nothing relevant.

Childhood: Parents happily married, kind and loving. Both were very conscientious people and concerned about what the neighbours thought. Mother was a worrier, especially about the children and money. Both had children by previous marriages. At the time of the patient's birth these were: sister, 16 years; sister, 14 years; sister, 13 years; brother, 11 years; and sister, 9 years. The patient was the first child of the marriage, followed by sisters 13 months and 5 years younger. Thus rather a lot of people to take care of her. Parents died when patient was 15 years, she then ran the home for the younger children.

School: 5 years. Happy, good mixer, enjoyed games, in A stream at secondary school.

Work: 14 years. Shop work, happy. 15 years, housewife. Has worked in shops and factories since. Now in a factory job which she liked until recently when her symptoms troubled her at work.

Sex: Plenty of boyfriends. Married age 19 years, happy marriage, sexually satisfactory. One daughter died aged 2 years in 1951. Son aged 20 years is well and happy. Own house, enough money, both in work, no problems

Medication: Triptafen and Valium (both withdrawn before discharge).

Patient's comments after 4 months' treatment

"I have suffered for many years with nerve trouble, first becoming apparent in 1951. In that year I had depression, panics, anxiety following the death of my little daughter aged 2 years. My doctor prescribed tablets for me which I took for about 2 years. In July 1964 I had an hysterectomy operation, in October that year I was admitted to the psychiatric hospital suffering acute depression, anxiety and cancerphobia. I was given eight ECT and discharged in early December. Each month I attended the clinic. For about 3 months I felt better, then my condition began to go worse again. I was again admitted, although I was not worrying about cancer, I was very depressed and suffering anxiety and feelings of panic. I was given a further twelve ECT. After having this treatment I was no better. I discharged myself from the hospital and started a 2-year struggle to overcome panics, vomiting, sleepless nights and anxiety. During these two years I attended the clinic once a month. In 1971 my doctor prescribed Triptafen and Valium because I was feeling that my throat was closing up, tension and panic. I was taking these tablets on and off until 1976. My condition became worse again in 1977. I could not cope with the panic, anxiety and depression. My doctor arranged for me to see Dr Bovill who advised me to have group psychotherapy and relaxation exercises. I have attended both for 16 weeks.

I am much better now. I have learned how to accept neurosis and not be afraid of it. I have learned how to cope with panics and, most of all, to understand neurosis. The anxiety and depression are gone, mainly I think because now I do understand, I do accept it and I am no longer afraid. My attending group therapy and discussing the way that one feels, and realizing that each person attending the group has a problem just as much as you do, helps tremendously. I wish I had known about psychotherapy years ago.''

Patient's comments added at completion of treatment

''I have now attended group psychotherapy for 13 months having been troubled with neurosis for more than 20 years. I am very pleased to say that I am now much better. I think the main reason for this is because I found out the cause of the neurosis and learned to understand it and accept it. Meeting people in the group each week and hearing them speak out about their fears also helped me because most of their fears were the same as mine, and so it was a comfort to me to be able to speak out about my fears and not be ashamed of them, as I had been in the past. I found within the group there was a sort of feeling of, 'We'll all try and help each other'.

Psychotherapy has helped me a lot and I can only say how grateful I am to the people who have worked to make psychotherapy treatment possible for me.''

[Letter a year after discharge.] ''I am still very well.''

Author's note

At the time of referral it was noted that:

(1) Her mother worried exceptionally about the children. It was thus likely that the patient would have learned to worry exceptionally about her own health and her children. Precipitating factors of neurotic episodes were: (a) death of a child, (b) hysterectomy, (c) arthritis.

(2) Her parents were conscientiously concerned that their children should be respectable in the eyes of the neighbours. Psychiatric illness

is not respectable. Her shame and sense of foolishness is apparent, it had destroyed her job satisfaction, and her comment on her treatment clearly shows the importance to her of this facet of her neurosis. Understanding her condition and meeting others with the same condition alleviated her shame.

(3) The habit of dependence was likely to have taught her by her five much older siblings, this being one of the ways in which older children are likely to establish their superiority over younger children. In a less happy home it might take the form of bullying interference against which the subject would rebel; but in an affectionate, closeknit family too much 'helping' of the first new baby for nine years was very likely. She states that she was much better after 16 weeks' treatment and she repeatedly attended a class saying that she was symptom-free and able to cope with symptoms should they recur. The therapist then suggested discharge. The patient would attend the next class in a relapsed state; she attended three different classes. Therapists suggested 'inadequate, dependent personality' as a diagnosis, but in the end she overcame her dependence on the therapist, her classmates and Triptafen. She withdrew the medication although she had an ample supply and, having managed on no medication for a few weeks, asked for her discharge.

(4) The term 'depression' occurs repeatedly in the history given by the patient and in her comments. During 13 months' attendance she never appeared depressed. This, of course, is due to a facet of her training in respectability, 'depression' being today the most socially acceptable euphemism for psychiatric illness. It is therefore always a mistake to believe the patient who says he or she is depressed unless and until he describes the symptoms of depression. Of course she was depressed following the death of her child but this does not account for anxiety symptoms lasting 2 years. She was endogenously depressed following hysterectomy, she was hypochondriacal and waking early then and only then; these symptoms responded to ECT × 8 and never recurred. But ECT × 12 was prescribed when, 6 months later, anxiety symptoms alone recurred. This common psychiatric behaviour is probably due to two causes. First, a failure to diagnose neurosis in the presence of a previous history of endogenous depression; second, if a diagnosis of neurosis is made, a frustrating sense of impotence in the absence of a known treatment for neurosis capable of application in the National Health Service climate. ECT is then prescribed in hope rather than in faith.

(5)   This patient had good parents. She was a happy child, well adjusted at school, socially, sexually and at work. It is important to appreciate that these circumstances do not necessarily preclude mistakes in the training for lifemanship which, if suitable circumstances later arise, will lead to neurotic symptoms. It is the exceptional circumstance of the child that it is important to note and evaluate.

That, in this case, was the fact of being the first baby for 9 years in the presence of five older siblings, four of them girls. In this situation all family training patterns would have been exaggerated as a result of the patient having seven teachers in respectability, worrying about children/health, conscientiousness and dependency. Her very presence as a pupil would have shielded the two younger ones from overtraining, at least to some degree.

Because it is impossible to criticize this patient's parents this case demonstrates the limitations and/or antitherapeutic results of attempting, through the written or spoken word, the mass education of parents in the mental welfare of children. Efforts in this direction render the goodwilling overanxious concerning child care while the badwilling are left untouched. Moreover, an overall negative result of these efforts has been, and still is, to cause a gross confusion in the minds of the public concerning the differentiation between the 'mad' and the bad. Hence, to name but two examples, some dead battered babies and some dead policemen. I offer no suggestions as to preventive medicine in the matter of neurosis, except to say, emphatically, that it is a matter of national importance and economy that treatment should be available for neurotics of or below child-rearing age.

PATIENT 4, MARRIED WOMAN, BORN 1945

Diagnosis: Anxiety state and intense sense of inferiority. Congenital chorea causes constant spilling of cups etc. and difficulty in writing.

Attendances: 20 in 1975–76, at age 30.

Complained of: Temper tantrums with husband and children aged 3 years and 1 year.

The following is an extract from an undated letter received soon after discharge:

"I said I would write and let you see by this letter that you and the group have done a lot for me . . . . I have now got the power to be happy once again as is all the family. This means a lot to a marriage and to me as I think you will agree.''

A further letter was received in 1979 saying she was well and happy.

PATIENT 5, MARRIED WOMAN, BORN 1947

Diagnosis: Anxiety neurosis.

Attendances: 17 in 1975, at age 28.

Complained of: Agoraphobia for 2½ years and frigidity of recent onset.

The following is an extract from an undated letter:

"I don't think I could have overcome my problems without your help . . . . Since leaving the group I have passed my driving test, something I have wanted to be able to do for a long time. You once said to me that when I had 'learned to cope with my nerves' I would pass, and I have proved you right.''

PATIENT 6, MARRIED WOMAN, BORN 1941

Attendances: 18 in 1976, at age 35.

Complained of: Worrying depressions and a suicidal attempt. Well until 10 years previously. Husband a heavy drinker, violent. Four children, age 16 years to 5 years.

The following is a letter received 1978.

"Just a few lines to let you know that I am now feeling fine. It is a long time since I last saw you, and I have gone through a lot since I last saw you. I will not go into detail because it is the same old story. Anyway on September 17th 1977, I arrived home from work, and an argument started, and I got a good thumping as usual. So I sent for the Police to have him put out of the house, and decided from then on there was no coming back. So I went to the Solicitor on the 19th September. I have now got my injunction, and will have my divorce, and everything settled by September this year. I have all my children but find it hard financially as he has not paid anything to the two young children since the day he left. I am waiting for the Court Order for maintenance. But now I feel great, and people keep telling me how well I look. I should have done it long ago when I think back that I tried to take my life through him, I must have been crazy. I should have got rid of him instead. Our household is all happier, and the atmosphere is great. If it had not been for you, and the other doctors at the groups I don't think I would be happy now because you all helped me to harden up and start to stick up for myself. And I have never forgot the advice you gave me, and it has all turned out for the best. Thank you very much hope you are well yourself and that your dogs are alright.''

PATIENT 7, MARRIED WOMAN, AGE 28

The woman who told this story was asked to write it for publication to illustrate the influence of the popular image of psychiatry and of relative pressure on the rate of failure-to-attend and dropout.

''On going to my GP suffering from headaches, depression and frequent bouts of crying I was sent to hospital for tests. The doctor believed that my heart was to blame because I was having much pain and many blackouts. The tests proved negative but my condition remained the same.

My marriage had broken up, my husband having left at my request. He had frequently beaten me up and repeatedly called me crazy or a headbanger, and he said I needed psychiatric treatment. At my fourth visit to the hospital the doctor advised me to see a psychiatrist. My first thought was that he too thought I was crazy. I went to pieces but agreed. I cried all the way back to work and, once there, went to see my welfare worker. She could see I was in a state and explained that the image most people have of psychiatrists is wrong, she said they were ordinary people and there to help. I still felt that I was going crazy and would be locked away as my husband had always said. You see, because I didn't understand, the word 'psychiatrist' frightened me to death, so I went through Hell for a month until I saw the consultant concerned.

Then things became clearer, I realized I was not crazy. I discovered that my condition was due to my rejection in childhood by my parents, so the rejection by my husband was too much for me to cope with on my own. I started group psychotherapy once a week, I still attend but now know that I am not crazy, that it was all because I didn't understand, I now know that it is the understanding that counts most. It's when people keep telling you that you are crazy, then the doctor suggests a psychiatrist, that you soon believe that you are mad.

I am very thankful for psychotherapy, it has helped me and many other people get well due to it too. It does take time but it's worth it even if it does take time and, sometimes, very many sessions.''

PATIENT 8, MARRIED PROFESSIONAL WOMAN, BORN 1940

Diagnosis: Hysteria;

Attendances: 20, March to December 1974.

"I write this as an 'ex' patient, I strongly emphasize that 'ex', because on no account do I wish to get back into the state I was in a few years ago.

I think that the moment the patient gets into serious difficulties is when he becomes afraid of the symptoms/sensations produced by tension and stress, by allowing himself to become afraid he puts himself into a circle of fear–adrenalin–fear. The more fear, the more adrenalin, the more sensations of fear.

How vividly I remember those intense panic attacks, how I was virtually rooted to the spot, unable to move for fear I was about to die. The palpitations, when one's heart feels about to burst, the breathlessness, the tight feeling, like a great weight on one's chest, the endless miserable list of dizziness, sweating hands, jelly legs, churning stomach, the strange tricks of vision, the feelings of unreality as if walking in a nightmare, the pattern of continuous fear and tension. I mention this list of symptoms because I think once a patient realizes that these feelings (and that is all they amount to, mere feelings) are not unique to him alone, and that others too have trod this miserable path, he has taken the first step along the path to recovery. I am sure I spent months convinced that no-one had suffered as I was doing.

As the attacks and symptoms get worse, the patient really begins to feel sorry for himself, terrified of being alone, in case of an attack and on the other hand afraid to be with others in case he has an attack and makes a fool of himself. I myself fought a losing battle through four different doctors (I simply could not get it into my head that I was suffering from the symptoms of fear, rather than 'heart attacks' as I was convinced my symptoms were). I could paper a room with all the electrocardiograph readings I had taken. My own life and that of my poor family was a disaster.

Then in 1974 I started group therapy classes (just imagine there were actually others wandering God's earth in the same state as myself!!) By December 1974 after 21 therapy sessions I was discharged, with a firm handshake, and a permanent invitation to return to the clinic, should I ever want to. I was ready to face any adversity. Little did I realize how well I had been taught to cope with life. At the beginning of 1975 I was in a big city hospital with, as was then diagnosed, Hodgkins Disease (which is cancer of the lymphatic system). On the same day as my admittance to hospital, I had another matter to attend to, the funeral of my mother, who had committed suicide by drowning.

During all of this time, of the trauma of my mother's death, of complicated tests and X-rays, of the looming up of major surgery, of prolonged and drastic radium treatment, I literally never turned a hair. I was so calm and faced the bleak future with utter acceptance – me – who could not face an attack of palpitations or a little dizziness without upsetting the entire health service. Now, that I had something real to worry about, something very real and very frightening, I could cope with it all.

After three gruelling weeks in hospital, it was unbelievably announced that a wrong diagnosis had been made, and that I had a blood disorder by the incredible name of toxoplasmosis.

A year later my only brother suffered a severe stroke at the age of 30 years. Today he is a total and helpless cripple, and I still haven't turned a hair. My lesson was well taught and very well tested out.

I realize even now the 'bogey' of anxiety/nerves can return occasionally. Sometimes after a period of stress or an upset of some kind or another the old familiar sensations can return, but it's because they are old and familiar that they are not so frightening anymore. It is when fear strikes first that it strikes hardest. I have learnt to wait quietly and calmly, and I know these periods will pass, because I have been taught the way out. I know that all the feelings no matter how frightening will go away.

I firmly believe that by the therapy I received I was shown the dark and difficult path to recovery; it was hard work, very hard work. I know the complicated way out of the maze now and I am at the top of the difficult climb, with reassurance that should I ever stumble and fall there are still those people who helped me up, and most important showed me how to stay up when I fell before . . . . 1979.''

Sought further treatment, seen four times briefly, individually, then again discharged.

Author's note

A common behaviour pattern of the hysterical personality comes out clearly in this account, in that this patient was at her best in the presence of real disaster and emergency. While coping with such circumstances she enjoyed the inward sense of importance she lacked ordinarily; she was thus obtaining primary gain as opposed to secondary gain. She admitted playing to the gallery with 'beautiful indifference' when she was believed to be dying, but this is harmless and certainly preferable to demonstrations of agony of mind at the prospect of death. Such behaviour as hers is to be expected in those with inborn histrionic characteristics when they find themselves in a dramatic situation, so condemnation is certainly not appropriate. It is the humdrum 'common round and daily task' which such personalities find hard to tolerate.

When she relapsed I considered that these aspects of her case would be better discussed individually than in a group, as I think they were.

10

Therapists' Comments

MR J. D. KENINGHAM, SCHOOLTEACHER

When the family business broke down I decided to support my family
by teaching. I entered teacher training college at the age of 40 and then
started to suffer fear symptoms of which nausea was the worst. These
occurred in any social situation, lecture halls, students' lounge and on
public transport. Having previously been treated for cancer I at first
thought my symptoms due to a recurrence and, though investigations
were negative, I still worried lest the doctors should have missed something.

I was referred to a psychiatrist who prescribed tranquillisers. On
these I felt anxious and ill as before but also half doped, yonderly and
exhausted. Intensive relaxation was tried and I soon became expert at
lying on the floor in a state of limp unreality but felt no better in the
outer world. Desensitization therapy was next prescribed, this first
entailed building up a hierarchy of symptom-invoking situations with
the therapist. Starting with a minor stress situation, in my case buying
a cup of coffee in the students' lounge, building up to sitations with
which I felt I could not cope at all. With the therapist I would relax, he
would suggest the minor stress situation which automatically caused
me to tense up, he instructed 'relax', when I had done so he would
again suggest the stress situation causing tension again, and so on *ad
nauseum*.

When I had been under one or other treatment for about 2 years I
became able to buy what must have been the most expensive cup of coffee in Britain. Given time I might have overcome each situation this.

way but life would not have been long enough. The psychiatrist decided that I had had my share of NHS treatment so I should pull myself together and come back in 6 months if I wanted to.

By then I had completed my teacher training and started to teach but, finding myself unable to cope with a class while suffering panic, I had gone sick under my GP. No diagnosis or explanation for my condition had been given me, I was unable to function normally at work or in social situations, the advice to pull myself together inferred that I was responsible for my condition and/or wasn't trying; this added a sense of guilt without telling me how to overcome my 'fault'. Then I began to wonder whether I were going mad. So, one way and another, I was getting pretty desperate when, some months later, my GP said he had read an article on a 'cure' for my condition written by a psychiatrist in Burnley, 30 miles away. I clutched at this straw, an appointment was made and, very nervously, I kept it.

I was utterly staggered to find that as I described my feelings the doctor would interject with such comments as, 'And I suppose you feel.... I know, I have been like that myself'. For the first time someone seemed to understand how I was feeling and I no longer felt myself to be the only person in the world to suffer this type of affliction.

The effort required to get to my first group meeting was very great as all my symptoms got in on the act. Tension resulting from sitting in the group was unbelievable until another patient began to talk; I then again discovered that I was not alone in my affliction, this enabled me to relax a bit and take in some points. I drove home with the feeling that perhaps, at last, something could be done for me as others seemed to be in much the same state as myself, though I was convinced that they were not as 'ill' as I. I was also impressed, as a teacher, with the manner in which the group had been conducted. It was very much like a tutorial in college, the accounts and observation of each person in turn being probed, questioned and thrown about, the individual being led to answer his own questions.

In the group I was told that my problems were really in the nature of bad habits. It was explained to me how one can be led in early life into certain ways of thinking about one's self – about one's capabilities and one's value as an individual, and how this can become an incorrect personal assessment of oneself. I was told of the multitude of ways in which we can react to this incorrect assessment and training as a defensive measure. It was made clear how all this becomes 'habit' and is no longer 'thought out' – one just reacts in that way. In other words I was led from a very inward, subjective, view of myself and my problems to a more rational, objective view. I was helped to 'stand outside myself' in order to view my situation more clearly.

During the course of the groups I was given tasks to do, such as to gently take a ride on a bus (one stop only) and have a panic attack deliberately. I was taught how to accept a panic attack without 'fear of the fear', to expect the attack and cope with it realizing that it wouldn't kill me, nor was it the end of the world.

This, of course, is Desensitization Therapy –but with a difference. I now had some insight into what the panic attack was. I began to see a 'cause-and-effect' situation. I began to understand fear and anxiety and started to realize the physical effects these had upon me. I began to realize that the worst part of an attack was the fear of the attack itself.

What now became important was the way I began to cope with the attacks, and the way I accepted them. I began to develop an entirely new attitude towards them.

I now found that the relaxation techniques I had learned during my previous treatment were very useful. I began to see that just as I had automatic reactions of thought, I also had automatic reactions of physical muscular tension. I found that I was able to be objective enough to recognize the muscular tensions brought on by stress situations and that I was able to practise relaxation techniques in order to combat these to some effect during a panic attack. This helped with my 'nausea' problem.

I now found that instead of spending nearly all my time in negative thoughts of 'fear and anxiety' I spend most of my time 'thinking through' my earlier life and how this had brought about the situation I was now in.

I had always considered that my upbringing had been excellent – almost privileged, very secure and 'middle-class'. But now I began to see that in no way had I been allowed to become 'me'. I had been grossly overprotected and had never been allowed to learn how to deal with the rough and tumble of real life. The aspiration and expectations put upon me had been rigidly imposed, and had never taken into account my natural abilities and desires, or my shortcomings and genuine dislikes. I had been programmed rather like a computer. Also, I had not been helped to come to an understanding and acceptance of my physical self, particularly with regard to my sexuality.

Whilst I do not consider it necessary to recount fully the intricate web of this 'thinking' I had now started to occupy myself with, I feel that some examples are important to show a 'model' of the way that directed group therapy does start a 'reconstructive thought process' in the patient's mind.

I must make the point that these 'reconstructing thoughts' only started after I had been taught how to deal with the panic attacks in a positive way, freed from some of the fear that they had previously engendered. I had also been given a basic understanding of automatic learned reaction to stimuli (Pavlov's dogs, for instance) and a vague understanding as to how the individual can come to a personal incorrect assessment of himself upon which his very thought and reaction is based, causing confusion, stress and undesirable defensive activity to occur entirely automatically.

As my nausea was perhaps the most annoying of my symptoms, if not perhaps as limiting as my 'social contact' problems, this was the first subject of my thinking. I began to remember past occasions in my life when it had occurred. I remembered feeling sick before going to parties and dances, and began to realize that these had always been stressful to me because of my shyness and reticence in company. As memories gradually trickled into my mind, I remembered that up to the age of 8 I had always enjoyed parties in spite of my shyness. I remembered that at the age of 8 I was sent to a large elite grammar school, and that I very quickly became a 'school refuser'. This must have caused my parents great worry, as I remembered that I had been sent to some sort of educational psychologist because of this. Although this consultation had no results whatsoever when I was 8 that I can remember, I now started to think and wonder why I had found the change to a new school so frightening. I now remembered that the way I used to get out of going to school regularly was by being sick!

There it was! I had regularly used the symptom that I was now unable to get rid of, as a useful tool to get me out of a recurrent stress situation.

But why was the school situation so frightening? At last a memory came into my mind. I rememebered the lavatory arrangements at the school with their open urinals, and the fear that these used to give me. I remembered being terrified of exposing my body in front of others either in a urinal, or in the changing rooms for gymnastics or games. I must have been physically advanced for my age as I used to obtain regular and prolonged erections of the penis at this time, and I remembered that this used to terrify me. I had certainly never been told that boys did get erections, and I thought that there must be something wrong with me.

Memories kept returning, and I remembered quite clearly an incident that occurred when I was about 3 years old, which I am quite certain I had not thought about consciously since it had occurred.

My bedroom was being decorated, and my bed had been put in my parent's room. That night I woke up after my parents had gone to bed in order to urinate. I remembered getting the chamberpot from under the bed, and then being unable to pass water because I had an erection. My mother, on seeing this, scolded me severely and told me that this had occurred because I must have been 'playing with myself'.

This appears to have been the only 'training' I ever received as a young child regarding the natural functions of the male reproductive organs!

I now began to think that perhaps this grossly inadequate training about my sexuality at that early age was the reason that I was quite unable as a teenager to 'go out with girls', because of my great fear of them (they caused the dreaded erections).

Then out of the blue came another memory. I was 5 years old and had just started school at a private kindergarten. I remembered going home one day and announcing that I had invited a friend home for tea the next day. My parents were very pleased at first and asked who the friend was. I told them that it was a girl called Jean. It appeared that the roof fell in! My parents were furious and told me in no uncertain terms that 'little boys *did not* play with little girls!'

There were many other aspects that I was led to probe. Why was it that I had always been so reticent and shy about using what talents I had? I had started to play the piano at an early age and was quite promising, as I loved music. But I had never been able to play in front of anyone other than my greatly loved piano teacher – whom I still think of as a wonderful person. (She seemed to have accepted me 'as I was').

Parental attitudes to my pianistic efforts appear to have been greatly encouraging, but I remembered that if I were to indulge in playing anything other than my 'set pieces', or to extemporize, which I loved to do, I would be firmly 'guided back to the right path' and told to 'play properly'.

I remembered being about 10 years old and having secretly obtained the music of the 'Warsaw Concerto'. This was kept secret from my parents and teacher because it was *infra dig*. One day I took this music into the music room at school before school began and was struggling through it on the school piano, when the school music master walked in . . . . The piano *was not* for grotty little schoolboys to play, and I received a detention for my efforts.

I remembered being about 6 and finding two old wooden planks in the garage at home. I nailed these together in a cross-formation. This was an aeroplane, and I held it happily on my shoulder and ran round to the garden where my parents were sitting in order to show them my creation. My father was horrified that I had produced such a badly made and ill-conceived model. He took it from me and chopped it up with an axe. He then gave me the small pieces of wood from the wreck of my plane and told me to try again and do better this time. Under his direction a new aeroplane was made, and it was much better than the first, but it wasn't half so much fun, and it wasn't 'mine'.

Another incident which came back to me very clearly shows that even at a very early age one has already come to set conclusions about oneself. I would have been about 7 years old, and was reassembling my fairy-cycle which I had taken to pieces. I was totally 'wrapped up' in reassembling the bike and was unaware of anyone watching me. As I struggled with the various parts I was talking aloud to myself: 'this bit goes on here, then that bit will fasten to that and then. . . .' My mother had been watching and listening. She told me that 'only mad people talked to themselves'. I remembered the great hurt of this remark, as I frequently indulged in 'thinking aloud' when alone. As I did this, then perhaps I was mad, I thought. This remark made by my mother seemed to be confirmation of ideas which were already planted in my mind at that time, ideas which could have only come from the experiences I had had at an even earlier age.

This remark about 'mad people talking to themselves' had stuck as a sore in my mind, and I now remembered travelling to school on the bus. I remembered sitting in the bus and dreaming either of things I was going to do, or just fantasizing. I remembered how ashamed I felt of these thoughts, particularly the fantasies, if another passenger should happen to look at me. I remembered feeling certain that I had been unconsciously talking aloud, and I would then sit tensely on the bus trying my hardest not to think of anything at all because of the 'shame' I felt about my thoughts. Eventually this became so bad that I conceived the idea that everyone else in the world except myself had another sense, akin perhaps to telepathy or mind reading, and that I did not even have the privacy of my own thoughts.

Here then, was one reason for my present 'stress situation' on buses and trains, although I had completely forgotten these early thoughts from childhood up till my period of 'reconstructive thinking'.

These examples show just some of the ways in which the mind is capable of working and recalling past, hurtful incidents long since consciously forgotten. One is now able to view these painful remembrances in an objective 'adult' way and realize the 'lie' behind the many factors which had caused this early hurt. One also sees how these are still causing reactions to take place entirely without one's conscious knowledge.

Reading through the above selections of 'remembrances' there appears to be a lack of cohesiveness, as only isolated memories are quoted. However it must be realized that this 'thinking' becomes almost a full-time occupation for one's waking hours, and that in fact a definite continuity is arrived at, and a clear picture presents itself to one.

As I started on this period of 'reconstructive thinking' during my waking hours, I found that my sleep was busy in dreams connected with my thinking.

I cannot remember many of these dreams now, although at the time they remained in my memory when I awoke. I can, however, remember a few, and will quote two in order to show the progression made.

My first dreams on beginning my treatment were all much about the same subject. Morbid dreams of death, graves, rotting human bodies, situations in which to my horror I was compelled to be.

One such was follows:

I was in a great church full of people whom I did not know. It was my Grandmother's funeral. The coffin was brought in and placed at the front of the church. I was sitting at the back. The people in the church took no notice of the entry of the coffin. Suddenly, my aunt stood up and commanded me to go to the front, open the coffin and kiss my Grandmother's corpse. I was filled with revulsion and horror, but recognized the command as being absolute and indisputable. Nobody in the congregation took the slightest notice of the command, or seemed to be aware of the horror it presented to me – just a sea of disinterested faces.

As my 'reconstructive thinking' progressed I began to have happier dreams, with a degree of optimism and occasionally even of feelings of joy.

Towards the end of my treatment I had a dream which was immensely relieving and satisfying to me:

A friend and myself had been out for a 'night on the town'. We were walking home in the small hours along the main street of the town, with shops on either side, when I saw a shop window full of display figures all dressed up in very official morning suits and top hats. I picked up a brick, threw it through the window, climbed in and urinated on the figures.

These dreams were subjects for me to talk about in the group sessions. I understood these dreams as follows, and gave these 'interpretations' to the group with the help of the therapist:

In the dream of the funeral I was shown how I was dominated by family influences, seen in the form of indisputable commands. It showed me that I was not able to act in a way that was 'of me'. I always acquiesced, against my natural desires, to these standards of behaviour and values which were set, and seen as being 'correct and proper', although I really felt them to be anathema to me. I was also shown, by the figures of the disinterested congregation, a picture of what happened throughout my life when my problems and desires were shown to others – no help and no interest.

In the second dream I realized that my 'reconstructive thinking' had led me to a point where I was beginning to gain freedom from this authority, and I was shown graphically how I was now able to 'piss on the figures of respectability and correct behaviour', and so begin to destroy the tyrannical hold that these had had over the totality of my life.

The progress in my thinking was monitored during group sessions, although only a fraction of what went on in my thinking was discussed. This was sufficient to guide me to do the 'spadework' on my own.

Perhaps, if I had been able to have a really competent full deep psychoanalysis I should eventually have come to much the same understanding of myself as I did through the group and my own thinking. However, I dread to think of the time that this would have taken, or the cost that it would have involved.

The statistics of the group show an average of 8 hours/patient/therapist time! It would be interesting to make an assessment of the time spent by the patient working through his problem – many hundreds of hours, I am certain! But because of the support and guidance obtained in the directed group these hundreds of hours are used effectively, leading forwards towards freedom from the root causes of the problems, and not negatively centred around the neurotic symptoms and the guilt, feelings of inferiority, fear and confusion that would otherwise be occupying the patient's thoughts.

At this point several observations about the running and conduct of the group must be made.

I must stress the intensity of agony, despair and confusion that gross neurotic symptoms bring to both the sufferer and to his family and friends. I find it almost impossible to put this suffering onto paper in any really meaningful way, but those of us who have experienced it will agree that it is far worse than any purely physical pain, possibly because it cannot be expressed clearly to others, and certainly because neither the sufferer nor those he tries to confide in understand what it is all about. There is a sense of loneliness and misery with neurosis which I can only describe as worse than death, possibly better described as 'hell'.

The 'group situation' immediately relieves a considerable amount of this loneliness. One finds that this 'hell' contains others, and this is initially immensely comforting. This could however lead to a state of mutual sympathy, and could cause a state where the people in the group wallowed together with ever-increasing cries of agony and woe.

This the directed group does not allow. Firstly, the therapist sees to it that although initial sympathy is shown to the new patient, after a very short time only understanding and empathy are allowed. Secondly, as the group is ongoing there are always members who have advanced sufficiently to be able to say 'Yes, I *was* like that, but now . . .', which lead the new member forward. Thus a state of affairs exists where 'if he can do it, so can I'.

The 'tutorial' form of the group in which the therapist directs discussion to one patient at a time has many other points in its favour.

Firstly, it is possible to avoid particularly voluble members 'hogging' the time available.

Secondly, it is easier to get a particularly shy or reticent member to join in by directing questions to him.

Thirdly, I found that it was much easier to absorb ideas when the therapist was directing his attention to another member. The nature of the neurotic is such that he often can go 'blank' when being talked to. By this I do not mean that he is unable to converse reasonably (although sometimes he does have difficulty), but rather that what is being said does not fully register with him. This is due to his general tenseness, and the universal wish on the neurotic's part to please. He just cannot say 'no', or argue a point. However, when he is listening as a third party to another member and the therapist discussing some point, a sort of 'rebound effect' or echo situation takes place. He is able to sit and listen, and to accept or reject points made without directly stating that he had accepted or rejected them. More often than not, this gives the listening member some point with which to start his own discussion with the therapist.

Since becoming a therapist myself I have heard these questions from several of the observers who come to 'sit in' on our group sessions: 'What happens if the therapist makes a wrong suggestion?' 'What about the morality of making pointed suggestions to patients?'

Because I have been a group member myself I am quite happy about these points. It really doesn't matter. One of the objects of the group is to start new thought processes in the patient's mind, and even an incorrect suggestion is capable of doing this. A neurotic is not 'mad', nor is he really incapable of knowing 'right' from 'wrong' even if sometimes he seems to be. Each individual seems quite capable of inwardly rejecting 'wrong' suggestions, a sort of inbuilt 'safety system'.

Sometimes a 'wrong' suggestion can bear more fruit than a 'right' one, in that it leads the patient to the 'right' answer from inside himself – far more valuable than having it spelled out for him.

A further question sometimes asked by observers is 'Does the patient's intelligence quotient, educational background or ability to verbalize problems have any bearing upon the patient's ability to be effective with his 'reconstructive thinking?'

The 'reconstructive thinking' process is not restricted to any particular type of neurotic manifestation, nor is it the prerogative of those with higher than average IQs or educational standards. It is seen in the groups that this type of thinking takes place with any neurotic patient who is motivated to begin, regardless of educational background or IQ (from about 80 +). This motivation to begin 'reconstructive thinking' is given to the patient in the group both by the 'leading' of the therapist, and even more importantly, by the concrete example of other members of the group who are already occupying themselves in this way.

Another question sometimes asked, usually by patients themselves, is: 'Does not this probing into parent/child relationships cause great problems of domestic disharmony, and great feelings of resentment against parents who may well be seen as the cause of the patient's suffering?'

Again, I am quite happy about this. Sometimes a patient will display great anger towards a parent, but more often the patient sees that whatever harmful or incorrect treatment they have received from their parents, it was done with 'good intent' on the parents' part. Sometimes patients can see that the way they have been treated has much to do with their parents' own neurotic problems, which had never been recognized, and can see a case of 'the sins of the fathers being handed down unto the third and fourth generation'. To use another Biblical quote, they are able to say 'forgive them, for they know not what they do'.

Whatever way the patient sees and reacts to this situation does not matter in the long run, as it is imperative that the whole complex problem of parent/child relationships is faced and understood in some depth. Most patients will eventually tell of greatly improved relationships inside their family, including relationships with parents, because of their own sudden increase in 'maturity'.

The 'tutorial' nature of the group has another valuable point in its favour. Each member is always addressed by his surname – Mr Brown, Mrs Smith. The groups, although friendly and open never take on a 'social get-together' aspect. These two factors together are important, as they help the patient to see himself as a person of 'standing' or value, and the group as a 'real' and valid experience in worldly terms.

If 'desensitization' is set in an artificial situation, it loses its 'reality'. It is not truly of the real world into which the neurotic is trying to find a secure foothold. Also if a therapist were to get too 'familiar' it would lead firstly to dependence (transference to a degree not desired) and also, strangely, it would increase the 'them' (above) and 'us' (below) situation, which these groups avoid at all costs.

Any contrived 'social group activity' would immediately be seen by the patient as being 'unreal' and set up for him. This would lead directly to the feeling that, first, he was being manipulated by others – again – and second, that he was such a 'poor fish' that it was necessary to have 'pretend' situations rather than real ones because that was all he was fit for, or worth.

It must be seen in the group that each person is esteemed as an individual of worth in order that he may start to esteem himself in the same way. At the same time the 'undeveloped' part of the group member is acknowledged (and accepted) and the patient is led to a situation where he can see the genuine 'adult' in himself, with full value and responsibility, and also the 'young child' part of himself, which he is helped to 'take by the hand and lead gently' into a more mature and realistic world.

It is necessary for a therapist to have a good understanding of neurosis; of course one way to get this is to have had disabling neurotic symptoms oneself. It is always easiest to help the patient who has the same symptoms as one had, but quite possible to treat patients presenting with different symptoms and problems because one is only leading the patient to do most of the work himself and supporting him while he does it.

An agoraphobic who is intent on overcoming his problems will work hard at desensitization and tell with pride of his success or with despair of his failure. The failures give the therapist the chance to teach him to go more deeply into why he failed, thus initiating reconstructive thinking. Those who progress well and easily on desensitization may not appear to think deeply or reconstruct at all, but on the groups they hear others doing so, thus it is probable that they absorb ideas and change attitudes to some degree.

Patients presenting with physical symptoms are often resentful of psychiatry, believing that they should be under medical treatment. I first suggest that they accept the physical symptoms and learn to live with them, I then try to lead them to think about their attitudes towards the symptoms and then about the situations which trigger them. Some patients have exaggerated fears of death, this too can be used as a starting point for reconstructive thinking.

Thus the therapist has to be flexible and prepared to use whatever material the patient offers to start the alteration of attitudes. He must be able to communicate in simple, easy words and nevertheless strike sparks off the patients. He must have enough self-assurance to be 'one of them', though one who has gone before. He must never give the impression of thinking himself superior nor a Solomon, but must often be prepared to say, 'I don't know'.

I work as a lay therapist because I find it fascinating. I was quite capable of living a full life when I completed treatment but teaching patients has added a depth to my understanding of myself and others; one never stops learning. Moreover, as a teacher, I think the most important thing one can do is to help an individual to come to an understanding of himself as unique and of value in the society in which he lives.

DR R. C. B. PETTIGREW, MB, ChB, DObst, RCOG,
General practitioner and clinical assistant in psychiatry

Neurotic illness accounts for a large percentage of the general practice workload, yet unfortunately remains the Cinderella of all clinical conditions. This could be ascribed to the lack of effective treatment available. The cornerstone of treatment up to the present time has been drug therapy, which is initiated either by the GP or the hospital psychiatrist. Psychoanalysis, once in fashion, has now been found to be far too time-consuming for the National Health Service, and who nowadays really believes that the root of all neurosis lies in childhood sexual fantasies? Behaviour therapy, more fashionable, and effective in certain conditions, circumvents the idea of experiential psychology and thus has pitfalls in treating the more deeprooted neurotic symptoms.

When I entered general practice I had experience in group therapy methods, and was fortunate to be in an area where a hospital psychiatrist was interested in the treatment of neurosis under the National Health Service. For this reason I decided to ascertain how tutorial therapy would help my own neurotic patients. I used certain criteria for referral and also for 'cure' after treatment.

When a patient came to surgery and presented with the psychic and somatic manifestations of anxiety, I explained to them what their symptoms signified. If the patient grasped the concept, I gave a long appointment at the end of evening surgery. A more detailed psychiatric history was taken and possible clues as to the genesis of neurosis were given. The purpose of the interview was (a) to exclude psychotic illness, and (b) to ensure that the patient was of such intelligence that he could understand basic principles. If, at the end of the interview, the patient demonstrated an eagerness to overcome his/her illness a referral was made for tutorial therapy. I make it a point always to explain to the patient what to expect from the psychiatrist and to erase the fear the patient has of being classified as 'mad'.

My criteria for a successful course of treatment are (a) a decrease in attendance at surgery with symptoms referrable to neurosis, (b) the abstention from psychotropic drugs, and (c) the ability of patients to cope with organic illness.

Over a period of 4 years 34 patients were referred and accepted for tutorial therapy. Of these, 15 completed their treatment and 19 failed to do so, having attended five sessions or less. Of those patients who completed treatment 13 (87 per cent) have remained free from neurotic symptoms of any kind and the remaining two have shown a definite reduction in surgery attendance though still using tranquillisers on a regular basis. Of course, when any of these patients attend surgery they are not always seen by myself; the notes to which I have referred before making these statements have often or sometimes been written by one of my two partners.

Despite the incomplete treatment of those who attended only one to five sessions, 77 per cent of those followed up, including alcoholics, showed considerable improvement. Possible explanations for improvement may be either the two long sessions for assessment and selection, one with myself and one with the psychiatrist, together with the patient's ability to grasp the basic concept of neurosis, or to the natural spontaneous resolution of the illness.

The main reasons for the high rate of failure to complete treatment were difficulties in travelling 10 to 12 miles to the hospital, with no public transport after treatment ended at 9 p.m., and the problem of finding a babysitter when the spouse was on either the evening or the night shift. Only a small percentage dropped out on account of failure to accept tutorial therapy; some might have rejected any form of group therapy.

These results have surpassed my own expectations of tutorial therapy as a method of treating neurosis.

In conclusion, one can say that this method of group therapy has a great deal to offer the busy GP. It gives an alternative form of therapy other than the use of drugs – thus reducing the enormous annual prescribing costs to the National Health Service. It immediately reduces the workload by obviating surgery attendances, the patient having the group rather than the GP for treating his condition. It not only teaches the patient to accept his neurosis, but also to accept illness as a whole. Possibly most important to the GP, it removes the ambivalence which, especially in the case of neurosis, can arise in the doctor/patient relationship.

DR A. SYED, MBBS DPH,
General practitioner and clinical assistant in psychiatry

I joined Dr Bovill four years ago as part of a team involved in psychotherapy. I had been trying to evolve a system of psychotherapy in general practice, but had found it extremely difficult to manage a group in the practice. However, after attending a few sessions with Dr Bovill, I realized that her technique of psychotherapy – teaching patients to cope with their neuroses – was, although not exactly alike, similar in many ways to my own.

This technique involves actually conditioning the patient to respond in a different way to his own emotional stimuli. We are all born with an 'inborn kit' of survival; when we are in danger certain hormones are produced which evoke the response of self-protection. The neurotic person, as a result of early conditioning, responds with fear to situations which others would not find frightening, so he or she cannot cope with normal situations. And in anxiety-evoking situations, such as examinations or interviews, the response of the neurotic is somewhat exaggerated, he becomes overanxious, this produces the symptoms of fear, such as palpitations, sweating and a feeling of choking. These people are helped only to a very small extent by drug therapy, they need an insight into their own problems and an understanding of the working of their survival kit. They also need reconditioning to cope with their own handicap.

I found this technique of teaching patients to cope with their handicap extremely helpful in general practice and I am certain that if a general practitioner could find 2 hours of his time per week he could treat ten to twelve neurotic patients in that time.

It is very rewarding to find that the success rate of treating these patients is excellent and I have no doubt in my mind that if a general practitioner selects his patients carefully, that is neurotics only, the success rate will be 70 to 80 per cent as shown in this book.

MR J. WOOD
Salesman

Alcoholics in the recently dried-out state must be brought to understand that stopping drinking is not enough, they must also rid themselves of their alcoholic thinking. Thus they must be deconditioned from negative emotional responses such as resentment, self-pity and remorse. Also their self-respect, which is seriously undermined, must be re-enforced. The task of the therapist is to train the alcoholic towards positive attitudes and towards the acceptance of life as it is. I have observed, therefore, that the alcoholic's rehabilitation parallels that of the neurotic, particularly the anxiety sufferer.

The therapist must always bear in mind that alcoholics are committed escapists, the early effectiveness of their escape route being perhaps their greatest tragedy. Tutorial therapy is of great value to the recovering alcoholic once he begins to understand that its purpose is to help him to stop running away from life.

The method lays primary emphasis on the acceptance of one's condition. This, again, is mandatory for alcoholics, who are legendary for their ability to rationalize their drinking. Alcohol will lead them into serious problems physically, mentally and socially, often to the degradation of themselves and others. But they will persist in the belief that they are driven to drink because of these problems. So the therapist must try to bring them to accept that alcoholism is an illness, that they have got it, that they crave alcohol because of it and drink from compulsion rather than rational decision.

Once this point of acceptance is reached tutorial therapy can proceed along the lines mentioned above, treating the alcoholic just as it treats the anxiety neurotic. The method's insistence on the acceptance of the possibility of disaster is of great importance to alcoholics, who must be conditioned to the belief that they can cope even in disaster, thereby diminishing the desire to escape: 'their worst day sober is better than their best day drunk'.

In my opinion alcoholics admitted for drying out should be encouraged to attend Alcoholics Anonymous, as they are at Burnley. I have noticed that AA encourages the cultivation of the open mind as a matter of survival and on a continuing basis. The resultant readiness for conceptual acceptance can only be of value to the therapist. But it has to be recognized that not all alcoholics relate well to AA, so though they should be encouraged to attend and to develop the habit of regular attendance, pressure should not be applied.

11

Administration, Selection and Management

As some of this chapter calls for considerable knowledge of psychiatry, it is directed primarily to medical readers.

The method is designed to provide, for comparatively large numbers, psychotherapy of a reasonable standard of efficiency with sufficient economy of medical time to render it acceptable in the peripheral staffing climate. Economy in time depends somewhat on organization.

ADMINISTRATION

At the time of writing the following was in effect.

Tutorial classes

Four are taken concurrently from 7–9 p.m. once a week, as this has been found to be most convenient for most patients and therapists. A large number attending together facilitates car-sharing. Five classes have sometimes been necessary, especially when there have been enough alcoholics to run a class specially for them.

Therapists

Each class has its own therapist; a consultant, two clinical assistants and one lay therapist take classes, a lay therapist in training takes a class in the event of holidays or illness. Lay therapists are voluntary workers, and only their travelling expenses are paid. Previously nurses have been trained as therapists, but nursing time has not been available in recent years.

Numbers and attendance

There are usually 50 patients, of both sexes, with the ratio of one man to two women; there are twelve to thirteen on the rolls of each class, and mean attendance is seven to eight. Absenteeism is largely due to the industrial shift system as it affects patients, spouses, 'chauffeurs' and babysitters.

History

A typed copy of each patient's history is in the class folder for the therapist's use. Particularly confidential material is excluded but, if relevant, it will be handed on to the therapist verbally.

Dropouts etc.

Patients who fail to attend for three consecutive weeks without communicating are visited by social workers, or community nurses if time allows, to ascertain the reason and offer a clinical appointment to discuss alternative treatment if appropriate.

Observers

Medical, nursing and ancillary workers who wish to study the method are welcomed, but not more than two are accepted in each class. If possible they attend three consecutive meetings of one class; they are introduced to the class but asked to take no part in the proceedings.

Selection

Following one consultant interview for history and assessment patients are accepted for immediate attendance at tutorials. They fall into three broad classifications:

(1) Those with confirmed neurotic diagnoses, including alcoholics.
(2) Those who, in the presence of unlimited psychotherapists, would be treated individually, in other words:

    (a) Those who feel themselves rejected by society and so integrate with a group with difficulty, if at all; these are often found amongst immigrants, homosexuals, the grossly overweight compulsive eaters and the personality-disordered.

    (b) Those who are on or beyond the borderline of the usual age-limits for acceptance for the treatment, which are 18–59 years. Patients aged 14–17 years occasionally used to be referred, and indeed a few integrated and benefited, but recently an adequate child guidance service was established. Occasionally a 60-year-old patient has seemed sufficiently flexible to stand a chance of benefiting, but such patients almost never integrate, indeed some in their 50s reject the method saying that it is shaming in the presence of younger people to admit the need for treatment.

Any of these kinds of people might integrate with a group of their own kind but do not present in sufficient numbers at any one time for such tactics to be practicable. Those that do not integrate usually drop out.

Consultant time is saved, some might say ruthlessly, by offering only a group method of psychotherapy to those who are likely to reject it. In reply I plead, 'The greatest good for the greatest number', and add that the offer is worth making because a few complete treatment and derive benefit. The traditional method of managing neurotics in the periphery, that is, occasional brief visits to a junior doctor's or clinical assistant's clinic for reassurance and prescriptions, is still available to those who reject the group method. Individual psychotherapy is offered when time is available.

(3) Those with doubtful diagnoses which include 'neurosis' are accepted for observation and provisionally for treatment, in those classes which are medically staffed. Patients under mistaken diagnosis may also be found as a result of observation in classes.

The flexibility of a system of several open groups running concurrently makes practicable and satisfactory the immediate acceptance of patients for treatment or observation. This immediacy is thought to be important in the treatment of neurosis and alcoholism. The advantage of having in operation a system which immediately provides 2 hours per week of medical observation for patients with doubtful diagnoses requires no comment.

The observation provided not only represents an economy in clinic time but is more efficient than the formal clinic appointment, because it is difficult to maintain 'cover' for 2 consecutive hours while in a group of people who are frankly discussing their symptoms and problems with the therapist. Thus the bizarre thoughts of the pseudo-neurotic schizophrenic, the morbid ruminations of the endogenous depressive and the irrelevant remarks of the early brain-damaged patient are more likely to be revealed in a tutorial than at a follow-up appointment.

Patients of borderline intelligence might be classified either among those unlikely to integrate or those accepted for observation. If they find themselves unable to follow the trend of a discussion they may drop out, or it may be the therapist who suggests alternative treatment. The intelligence test is not always a reliable guide. I have known a patient aged 58 with an IQ of 72, who had been housebound for 35 years, make a remarkable recovery to the point of starting a clothing club in her village. Admittedly such an event is very rare but once the tutorial system is operating nothing is lost by giving such patients the opportunity to benefit.

Thus observation at tutorials, results of investigations or review of records from elsewhere, may lead to the withdrawal of a patient from tutorial therapy and institution of treatment more suitable to the confirmed diagnosis.

It has been suggested that the withdrawal from tutorials of those found unsuited to the treatment, together with the disappearance of dropouts, could prove discouraging or disturbing to those likely to benefit from the treatment. In practice this does not appear to be so, perhaps because the session is being run like a class, with the therapist as focal point; or perhaps because, as in all open group methods, patients are continuously joining, being unavoidably absent, returning after absence, and, finally, being discharged. Moreover, classes accept observers without apparent change in the quality of the work done. In short, tutorials always have shifting populations so a few more absentees pass without comment.

A common excuse for failing to offer psychotherapy to neurotics is shortage of medical time, so no apology is needed for measures that make time available provided other patients receive their fair share. The inclusion of patients for observation in tutorials reduces consultant follow-up appointments in clinics, thus providing consultant time to practise psychotherapy, to be available after the weekly tutorial sessions to discuss problems with co-therapists, to teach trainees and discuss with observers, to see any patient giving cause for concern, or anyone who, having been treated by a lay therapist, is seeking discharge.

I never found it impossible to organize my time so that other patients received the attention they needed. I nearly always maintained my waiting list at about 3 weeks while seeing in a year about 300 new referrals and giving about 1000 follow-up appointments. I also saw suicidal attempts/demonstrations and other patients referred from the medical and surgical wards. An occasional acute emergency sent in by a general practitioner would also be fitted in, or perhaps a periodic case conference for non-accidental injury to children; a weekly ward round and one or two meetings in a month completed the programme. How this compares with the workload of consultants elsewhere I have no means of telling, but the point I am anxious to make is that my work for neurotics in no way deprived other patients because the method of psychotherapy is so economical in medical time.

REQUIREMENTS FOR TREATMENT BY TUTORIAL THERAPY

These are somewhat flexible but as a rule are as follows:

Age: 18–59 years.
Intelligence quotient: 70 + (Raven)
General health: adequate to carry out housewifely duties but excluding severe chronic or terminal disease.
Hearing: adequate to hear the spoken word with hearing aid if worn.
English: command of the language sufficient to understand and speak it freely.
Neurotic diagnosis: confirmed as a result of observation at tutorials.

I first laid down the basic requirements for acceptance for tutorial therapy when collecting patients for the controlled study (see appendices (a) and (b)); at the time I accepted all psychopaths and excluded all endogenous depressives. As a result of accepting all neurotics who fell within the requirements, I found that I knew of no criteria with which to assess who would do well or badly – patients who appeared near hopeless did remarkably well and vice versa. Subsequent experience has confirmed this observation, so all patients who fall within the requirements are accepted and left to select themselves.

DIAGNOSTIC LABELS

Those which might be attached to patients treated in tutorials are: anxiety neurosis, neurotic depression, phobia, hysteria, hypochondriasis, obsessional neurosis, anorexia nervosa, compulsive eating, soft drug dependence, alcoholism and minor degrees of personality disorder.

Affective psychosis

Patients with a previous history of this condition are accepted for treatment by tutorial therapy, if there is a history of neurotic symptoms of long standing which do not remit as do those of affective psychosis. Patients are accepted only when the affective psychosis is in remission and only in those tutorials that are medically staffed. They are first accepted for observation to ensure that the psychosis is not active and they are treated with caution because, if depression recurs during treatment, morbid guilt feelings might be aroused by a failure to persist in following instructions which, if unobserved, might contribute to suicide. Thus the aims in treating these patients for neurosis are limited but benefit has been seen to occur (see patient 3, Chapter 9).

Other psychoses and dementia

Patients with these diagnoses are *not* accepted for tutorial therapy. Group methods have, of course, been used for them with some success, by myself among many others, but the approach is social and supportive as opposed to the positive counselling and retraining designed for those handicapped by neurosis. Schizophrenics, accepted for observation in tutorials before confirmation of diagnosis, are seen to be quite unable to relate to the counsel offered, which is usually the first indication of the true diagnosis. Many authors have described this phenomenon as 'the glass wall'.

Psychopaths/personality-disordered/moral deficients

Those mildly affected are accepted for treatment and young patients showing pseudopsychopathy, common in adolescence, are freely accepted for treatment: but, as has already been said, the more mature though mildly affected do not usually integrate well in tutorials and usually drop out anyway.

Patients in tutorials develop strong fellow feelings. It was in my early days of using the method that I observed the danger which this could cause if more severely affected psychopaths were included in the groups. One such patient, having been invited to the home of a fellow patient, stole tranquillisers and money which were not returned. Another invited a fellow patient to bring her children for a drive in a 'borrowed' car and took them down the M1 at high speed without driving licence or, consequently, insurance. Another made an abortive attempt to blackmail myself, an experience which could have been very disturbing if directed toward a patient. I also observed that only those with very moderate degrees of personality disorder responded to the method at all.

Group methods of the interpatient discussion kind are, of course, used for personality-disordered patients, but again the approach is different from that of tutorial therapy.

Addicts

Alcoholics are accepted for treatment; usually they are hospitalized for 12 weeks, initially on the usual medications at the time of withdrawal and then on Abstem or Antabuse. Weekend leave is progressively extended, they attend weekly tutorials and are encouraged to attend Alcoholics Anonymous. Those that have employment can work from the hospital, the unemployed attend the Industrial Therapy Department. Alcoholics are encouraged to attend tutorials for at least a year. When enough have presented a class can be run specially for them, which they prefer, although they appear to do equally well in classes with other neurotics.

Hard drug addicts have not presented for treatment, and I would not be hopeful of success were they to do so. Patients who, as adolescents, experimented with drugs are, of course, commonly referred for other reasons. Dependency on soft drugs is fairly common; when patients are improving they can usually withdraw medication gradually as outpatients, but occasionally admission has been needed.

Anorexia nervosa

Patients suffering severely from this condition are treated initially as inpatients.

TREATMENTS GIVEN CONCURRENTLY WITH TUTORIAL THERAPY

Inpatient treatment

The controlled study was conducted on patients who all started treatment as inpatients, these being the only patients to whom I had access at the time. Subsequently the majority have been outpatients throughout treatment. In the year reviewed (excluding alcoholics) 85 per cent were outpatients throughout treatment.

Alcohol and drug addiction, and anorexia nervosa have been mentioned above. Those referred as a result of a suicidal attempt/demonstration are often admitted to a ward for a few days. The wards have also been used occasionally as temporary refuge for a battered wife, otherwise it is extremely rare for a purely neurotic patient under psychotherapy to become sufficiently distressed to need admission. Those with a history of affective psychosis who relapse into this condition are withdrawn from psychotherapy at least until remission has occurred, so such cases were not included in the 15 per cent hospitalized.

Psychotropic medication

This is almost never prescribed for purely neurotic patients, but patients are often used to medication before they are referred. They are advised to withdraw it gradually, with the explanation that it is important not to mask symptoms while under treatment and that no known medication will cure their symptoms, a fact that many already know. Purely neurotic patients are not discharged until it is certain that they have been taking no psychotropic medication at least for a few weeks, but usually for much longer.

Relaxation

The method used is that of Dr I. C. Martin, and tuition is given by nursing staff. A minority of patients attend and only 20 to 25 per cent attend often enough to benefit from the classes; but the service is worth providing because some assert that they gain great benefit. Many have already been taught relaxation either when pregnant or through yoga lessons. Some buy the tapes for home use.

Individual psychotherapy

The majority of patients receive no individual treatment after the initial interview and prefer class attendance. I believe Adler (1929) was the first to comment on the psychotherapeutic effect on an audience of hearing others being treated. I think this influences patients to prefer classes to individual treatment, as they often comment on the amount they learn while listening to the treatment of other patients.

All patients know that individual sessions are available on demand, either briefly with the class therapist after a class, or by appointment with myself in clinic time. These interviews are sparingly sought, as they are usually for the discussion of a matter too private for the class – perhaps sexual or illegal. One interview almost invariably suffices.

A few patients need some individual treatment. Some are too shy to face the class, and these I see individually two or three times until they have gained enough confidence to join my class; later they may be transferred to another class. Others may have been previously treated by individual psychotherapy; if this has failed to help them they may be less hopeful or trusting while being conditioned to expect individual attention. The comments of one such patient appear in Chapter 9 (patient 1). Two or three individual sessions usually suffice.

Patients sometimes seek single interviews with me because they feel they are not progressing, or not happy, in a certain tutorial class – perhaps they are not in empathy with the therapist, or perhaps a close neighbour, friend or relation is also a member of that class, which may be embarrassing. After discussion with the therapist transfer to another tutorial class is usually a satisfactory solution but sometimes a few individual sessions are needed.

In order to discourage attention-seeking, which may be a motive for seeking individual treatment, I usually give either brief appointments (15 minutes weekly), or long appointments (45 minutes weekly), for individual psychotherapy and insist that the patient also attend tutorials, making an exception in the case of the shy beginner.

A therapist also sometimes asks me to see a member of his class either because progress is not satisfactory or because he has doubts as to the diagnosis.

Sexual counselling

When indicated this is offered to patient and spouse together.

Improvement

Patients often seek advice as to whether they are yet ready for discharge or, if seeking discharge, can sometimes be persuaded to continue treatment a little longer if this seems desirable. The first question I ask is whether medication has been discontinued, and if so, when; no purely neurotic patient is encouraged to discontinue treatment until medication has been withdrawn for at least some weeks.

Defining improvement sufficient to warrant discharge, I readily include those who have learnt to manage their fear symptoms well enough to disregard them and live a normal life in spite of them. A patient who has learnt to tolerate neurotic symptoms and ignore them will enjoy a gradual reduction over a period, perhaps of years, and if disasters cause a recurrence of symptoms he will once again cope with them. But a patient whose symptoms suddenly disappear almost certainly owes this factor to environmental change for the better, so when a change for the worse occurs, so will the symptoms, and the patient will be no better able to cope with them than before.

I enquire therefore, searchingly, as to whether the patient is still getting symptoms, and whether he/she can cope with them. If not, is he seeking them in the way he used to get them formerly; if he is not doing this I suggest that he makes sure that he can cope with any symptoms before he seeks discharge.

Date of discharge

This is patient-determined but at the time of discharge the patient is assured of a welcome if he wishes to return. Sometimes the therapist may doubt whether the improvement is sufficient to warrant discharge but, if the patient presses to be discharged, his assessment of himself will be accepted in the interests of supporting his courage and independence.

Some observers have thought it undesirable to allow *patients* to determine the date of discharge. Admittedly an occasional patient seeks discharge too soon for social or domestic reasons that he thinks may not be acceptable to the therapist. He does this while relying on the promise of a welcome back when attendance will be more convenient to him. But nothing has been lost by agreeing with his wishes; if this had not been done he would probably have dropped out completely and then found it more difficult to seek further treatment.

There are also those who are overoptimistic in seeking discharge before they are ready, but they usually discover the error within a few weeks and return to complete treatment.

The promise of a welcome back at some later date is helpful to the patient in two ways. First, it makes it easier to seek discharge when he/she is ready for it as opposed to clinging to attendance. Second, post-discharge anxiety is allayed by the knowledge that a telephone call to the department will assure him a place in the next tutorial session, so the availability reduces the necessity to seek reassurance. This provision reduces mean attendances and early re-referrals, which amply compensates for the minor irritation, rather than inconvenience, caused by the very few patients who abuse the provision by seeking, in effect, temporary discharge for their own convenience.

Dependence on attendance

Provided the classes are well filled, receiving a steady stream of new referrals, very few neurotic patients without added complications continue treatment longer than therapists think necessary. Dependence does occasionally occur, usually among those whose circumstances (age or marital, for instance) make it difficult to find a social circle. For these the tutorial represents the social event of the week. This is more likely to occur with those who find integration difficult generally, but have integrated, at least to some extent, with a tutorial class, those suffering under the stigma of mental illness, which often includes those who have been treated as inpatients for affective psychosis, those with marital problems, and those who are somewhat physically disabled.

It is very noticeable that as soon as the pressure of new referrals is taken off the therapists the mean attendance rate per patient rises. Presumably therapists unconsciously influence patients to seek discharge as soon as they think them ready to do so, but only do this when they themselves are under the pressure of a full class. Thus there is danger of running underfilled classes because there is more likely to be a habit of dependency among patients who have continued treatment longer than is necessary.

Management of a class

All patients attending a class are required to speak at every class after the first one, but they are reminded that they may speak on anything, that a class is not to be regarded as a public confessional, so they are under no constraint to speak on matters they do not wish to discuss in public, and that the therapist leaves the choice of subject to them. They are advised not to come with a prepared speech, but to say whatever comes into their heads when they get to the class. In stressing this point I tell them of a patient who said initially that she could not think of anything to say. I advised her to say the first thing she thought of and she said, 'There is dust on that lampshade!' From that starting point she and I conversed, usefully I think, for 20 minutes, she being an obsessional personality!

The therapist needs to watch the time, as he has 2 hours to divide between, say, five to twelve patients, depending on the attendance that night. A small attendance can lead to valuable work being done by a few, whereas a large attendance can provide a useful and lively tutorial.

The great majority of conversation is between patient and therapist, but after each such conversation the therapist should ask the class for comments, which can be very valuable. Sometimes a discussion starts, and it is up to the therapist to allow it to continue only as long as it is useful and doesn't become irrelevant, nor seem to exclude certain patients who may not then have time to speak at all at that class.

In the early stages of treatment particularly, the patient is anxious to get and keep the ball in the therapist's court, because he believes that the latter will take away his troubles. He has to be gently but firmly persuaded to play the thinking game himself. For example:

Patient: When I go out of doors my stomach turns over and I feel sick.
Therapist: What do you think causes that?
Patient: Is it insecurity? [Beware of 'umbrella' words picked up from the mass media and only half understood.]
Therapist: What do you mean by insecurity?
Patient: Is it inferiority?
Therapist: Let's start again, your stomach turns over and you feel sick, what is likely to cause those feelings?

The therapist keeps at it until he gets back the word 'fear' – having said it himself it is probable that the patient will remember it (that fear was causing these symptoms had been explained when his history was taken). If the therapist can't get the word 'fear' from the patient he asks the class, and with any luck several people will give it to him, thus reminding the patient.

Having established in the patient's mind the simple cause of his discomfort, the therapist moves on towards its management:

Therapist: What do you think is the best way to go on when we are frightened?
Patient: Get out of the way.
Therapist: Of course that is often right, but do you think no soldiers should go into battles and no firemen should go into fires to rescue people?
Patient: I didn't mean it that way.
Therapist: I know you didn't. But how do you think soldiers and firemen manage their fears?
Patient: They just get on.
Therapist: That's right. So how do you think you might manage your fear?
Patient: If it is *just* fear, I suppose the same way.

The therapist then explains that the patient should go out every day for short periods only, until he gets used to his fear, awarding himself a medal for bravery every time he does it.

Patient: But what am I frightened *of*? [This is the topic for next week.]

Points arising from this conversation will probably come up during ensuing weeks, and may include:

(1)   Is it really only fear, or has he got cancer of the stomach?
(2)   If it is just fear then is he not a coward? [No! Define courage and cowardice.]
(3)   Of what is he frightened? [Criticism]
(4)   Why is he frightened of criticism? [Because small children, being dependent, are all frightened of criticism, frightened for their lives, and perhaps he had an overdose of it, so he has a poor opinion of himself and expects everyone to have too.]

(5)   Why has he been 'alright' until now if this trouble comes from early childhood? [Discuss the natural history of the condition including the trigger or precipitating factor and the adolescent upsurge of drive and confidence.]

(6)   He feels inferior and ashamed of feeling inferior. [Encourage the patient to accept both as being just bad habits, and stop trying to shake them off; he knows he is not inferior, and it's not his fault that he feels inferior, so accept the feelings as just 'one of those things'. He must concentrate on reminding himself that he isn't *inferior* in all things and will certainly never be *superior* in all things.]

Maintenance of a friendly, encouraging atmosphere is important; if the therapist enjoys the tutorial it is probable that the patients will also do so. But it is sometimes necessary to take a firm line with a patient, as occasionally one patient tries to take up far more than his fair share of the time, and, very rarely, one patient is verbally aggressive to another. It is commonly desirable to remind a patient of his contractual obligations to attend regularly for treatment and to carry out instructions with regard to desensitization. Firmness may also be helpful in a situation such as the following:

Patient (who has been attending for some six weeks): Why do I feel so frightened when I go into a shop? What am I frightened of?
Therapist: What have we taught you is the answer?
Patient: I don't know.
Therapist: I think you ought to know, I'm sure you've been taught it several times. Let us see if anyone else knows, who can tell him? [No answer is received.] Mrs X you are attending your 21st tutorial, so you have heard the answer to this question at least ten times, probably nearer twenty times, are you sure you don't know it? [Still no answer.] I am going to tell you all *again*, will you please try to nail it into your heads, there is no sense in coming here to be taught if you don't learn what you are taught. What you are afraid of is criticism, of other people's bad opinions of you.
Class (in chorus): Yes, of course!
Therapist: Will you please all tell me why it is that you find it so difficult to remember this, that it goes in one ear and out the other?

After a pause someone will say, 'It's because we don't want to believe it'. A useful discussion will follow in which the following points can be made: (a) Freudian forgetting; (b) there are always going to be some people who think badly of us, we have to accept that; (c) the importance of self-assessment; (d) the enormous importance of self-acceptance; (e) the importance of facing up to realities that we find unpleasant.

It may appear as if the only patients under treatment by this method are phobics, and in a sense that is true because, as stated in Chapter 1, hysteria, obsessionalism and addiction are methods of escape from fear. Certainly the anxiety neurotic with his phobias presents a simpler picture because he has not yet complicated it, but the underlying problem is the same for all patients − fear.

I always try to send everyone home happy, though I do not always succeed. If I have taken a rather firm line with a patient I try to say something encouraging and to his credit before the end of the class. When I say, 'It's time to finish now', I add, 'Are you all going to be all right till next week?' And I end with 'Goodbye, it's been nice to have you here, I'll look forward to seeing you next week'.

Starting a new class

The easy way, especially for the inexperienced therapist, is to treat three or four patients two or three times individually and, while doing so, 'sell' them the advantages of the group method. Then invite them all together to 'give it a try'. Having thus obtained a nucleus it is best to refer all but the very shy patients to the class as soon as the history is taken, so it is then accepted as being the normal method of treatment.

12

Review of a Year's Work

Some of this chapter, like some of the last, may be somewhat obscure to lay readers, for which I apologize.

On 1 April 1976 I started my last year before compulsory retirement from full-time consultancy in general psychiatry under the National Health Service. Since starting work at Burnley, 3 years before, I had always thought myself to be too busy to keep records of the work in tutorial therapy, such as would enable me to render a truly accurate account of the numbers and kinds of patients that we were passing over this psychotherapeutic conveyor belt. In the 3 years the system had built up to its full potential, a steady stream of patients was being referred, enough competent therapists had been recruited and trained – the system was running smoothly. Thus it was not only my last chance to obtain accurate records of a year's work in a district hospital under full-time work conditions, but also an ideal moment at which to begin doing so. In this chapter I offer the findings of that year of record-keeping.

At that time I could not have foreseen that I should be so fortunate as to be re-employed, part-time, for psychotherapy only, for some years ensuing. This has enabled me to see completed the treatment of all patients treated during that year, to arrange for all those who could be reached, among patients discharged during the year, to be followed up, informally, 1 or 2 years after discharge, and to search the records to enumerate re-referrals to the department. These findings also are included.

I hope that these figures may be of some use and interest to young colleagues who, like myself at the beginning of my career, may believe that psychotherapy is so time-consuming that it can only be offered to a selected few under National Health Service conditions. Concerning the efficacy of the method I refer them to the papers on the controlled study reprinted in appendices (a) and (b), and can only hope that young and open minds will reject the theory that research into the efficacy of psychotherapy is as impractical and improper as would be research into the efficacy of religion.

Table 1 Scope of the method. This table shows the numbers of patients seen at tutorials during the year 1.4.76 to 31.3.77, their categories, the numbers who completed treatment, together with their mean ages and attendances for treatment

Categories of neurotic patients 1 to 7	Seen at tutorials during the year 1.4.76 to 31.3.77			Completed treatment					
	In treatment on 1.4.76	Intake 1.4.76 to 31.3.77	Totals	1.4.76	1.4.77	1.4.78	Totals	Age	Attendances
	N	N	N	N	N	N	N	M	M
(1) With no added complications	25	57	82	42	23	5	70	35	25
(2) The same but lightly affected	1	8	9	9	0	0	9	28	3
(3) Unlikely to integrate in a group	1	9	10	3	1	0	4	40	31
(4) With concurrent organic disease	3	7	10	5	1	2	8	38	36
(5) With personality disorder	1	13	14	2	3	0	5	31	15
(6) With alcoholism	6	17	23	11	2	0	13	36	44
(7) With concurrent endogenous depression in remission	4	14	18	9	4	2	15	40	26
Found diagnostically unsuitable under observation	0	12	12						
Totals	41	137	178	81	34	9	124	36	26

N = number
M = mean or average

NOTES ON TABLE 1

Throughput

This is seen to be continuous; 41 patients were under treatment on 1.4.76 and 43 on 1.4.77. (It was a chance finding that these figures were low, as 50 attenders was usual).

Rate of turnover

All those seen at tutorials before 31.3.77 had been discharged before 31.3.79. Time in treatment can be estimated from the mean attendances: an average patient attends about 30 sessions in a year; as shown mean attendances were 26; mean months in treatments were found to be 9. Alcoholics are encouraged to attend for at least a year, preferably longer, but out of 109 non-alcoholic patients only eight attended for 20 months or more, 26 months being the longest attendance.

Categories

Patients are classified into seven categories with the intention of attempting to assess the suitability of the method to the different categories:

(1) Without added complications either psychiatric or of general health, but with neurotic disablement of some severity and duration.

(2) Without added complications but lightly affected. These attended only one to five sessions before seeking discharge, saying either that they were not bad enough to need treatment or that they were cured. Spontaneous recovery as a result of environmental change account for some of these 'cures'. The mean age was 28 years, and all but two were under age 30. Some people, especially the young, are influenced by features on the mass media or the comments of others to become needlessly anxious about their mental health. When assessed in clinic their need for treatment may be doubted, but further observation is thought wise. Exposure to fellow patient/therapist discussions in tutorials may convince such a patient that his concern is needless. The management of such patients illustrates the advantage of having in operation a system of open group therapy, but whether they can be regarded as having been treated is very doubtful.

(3) Unlikely to integrate in a group. These may be subdivided into two classes:

(a) Those in whom the precipitating factor of the neurotic illness was their sense of rejection by society – often immigrants, homosexuals or grossly overweight compulsive eaters.

(b) Those on the borderlines of the age-limits for tutorial therapy, these being 18–59 years, who often feel that they do not 'belong' in tutorials.

In an ideal world all in this category would be offered individual treatment.

(4) With concurrent organic disease of some severity. The minimum standard of general health required is that it should be adequate for all housewifely duties (men are included in the same standard). Patients with impaired general health fall into three classes:

(a) Those in whom the stresses of self-desensitization may exacerbate the organic condition, examples being heart failure, hypertension, asthma and peptic ulcers. For such patients aims must be limited because the therapist dare not apply the same pressures to them as he would to others. Patients are referred back to the clinic and discontinue tutorials if the organic condition worsens.

(b) Those with conditions which limit physical activity, examples being muscular dystrophy and arthritis. Such conditions offer too good a reason/excuse for failing to practise self-desensitization. On some, or most, days the organic condition may be found to be too severe to permit this activity.

(c) Those with socially embarrassing conditions such as congenital chorea and colostomy. The courage demanded of such patients to overcome social phobias is obviously greater than that demanded of others.

With these difficulties to overcome a high mean of attendances was to be expected, but the range of attendances was wide, the lowest being eleven and the highest 69.

(5) With personality disorder. (The old term, 'moral deficient', is both more descriptive and less ambiguous, in that some would describe all neurotics as being personality-disordered.) Only those less severely affected are accepted for tutorial therapy. These patients do not integrate well in tutorial classes, and my impression is that they find it difficult to relate to a group of people who are not 'taking the mickey' out of 'authority' in the person of the therapist. They rarely complete treatment.

(6) With alcoholism. These fall into two groups, those who use alcohol as a tranquilliser and those whose alcoholism resulted largely

from occupational hazard and habit. All are accepted for treatment but the former are more likely than the latter to complete treatment and respond.

Alcoholics are encouraged to attend for at least a year, preferably longer, hence their high mean attendance. They prefer to have a class to themselves and did so during the year under review, but when their numbers were insufficient to form a class they appeared to do equally well when treated together with other patients.

(7) With concurrent endogenous depression in remission. These are patients with longstanding neurotic symptoms which do not remit when the endogenous depression does so. Their response to the method is often not very good, but it is probably good enough to justify

Table 2 Acceptability of the method to the patient. This table shows the numbers of patients introduced to tutorial therapy during the year who did not complete treatment.

Categories of neurotic patients	Total intake 1.4.76 to 31.3.77	Not able to complete treatment	Able to complete treatment	Dropouts		Age	Attendances
	N	N	N	N	%	M	M
(1) With no added complications	57	7	50	5	10	25*	2
(2) The same but lightly affected	8	0	8	0	0		
(3) Unlikely to integrate in a group	9	0	9	6	66	29	2
(4) With concurrent organic disease	7	2	5	0	0		
(5) With personality disorder	13	2	11	7	64	30	2
(6) With alcoholism	17	3	14	7	50	35	5
(7) With concurrent endogenous depression in remission	14	0	14	3	21	35	8
Diagnostically unsuitable	12	12	0				
Totals	137	26	111	28	25	31	4

*indicates significant difference at 5 per cent between the age of dropouts and the age of those who completed treatment.

N = number
M = mean or average

their treatment. The comments of patient 3 in Chapter 9 are relevant in this context. These patients are included in classes taken by medical therapists so that relapse into endogenous depression does not go unnoticed.

Those patients found diagnostically unsuitable under observation, or with doubtful diagnoses are accepted for observation in tutorial classes under medical therapists.

During the year twelve patients were found unsuitable for tutorial therapy; their confirmed diagnoses were: one schizophrenic, two borderline subnormal, one brain-damaged, one hypomanic and seven in active endogenous depression. All were referred back to the clinic for more suitable treatment.

NOTES ON TABLE 2

Failed to attend

Of 153 patients assessed and offered tutorial therapy during the year sixteen failed to attend at all.

Unable to complete treatment

This was due to such causes as change of job, change of shift, moving away from the area, inadequacy of public transport for those resident at a distance, sometimes aggravated by pregnancy or poor general health, and inability to replace a lost babysitter.

Dropouts

This term is used to indicate rejection of the method and, in the absence of known adequate cause for failure to continue attendance, patients were classified in this way. It was not always possible for staff to visit patients who had stopped attending, so the figures for dropouts will err in the direction of being too high rather than too low.

Dr Pettigrew (GP) comments in Chapter 10 that some patients who failed to complete treatment have benefited to some extent. Two patients in category (1), who had attended respectively six and seven tutorials, but were then unable to continue attendance, stated that they had benefited from the classes. Experience of patients in category (2) suggests that, unless all who fail to seek formal discharge are visited, which they could not be, there will be undiscovered patients who have dropped out because they believe themselves to have received sufficient benefit. It is of note that the mean attendance of nine patients in category (2) was three tutorials (Table 1), while the mean attendance of 28 dropouts was four tutorials (Table 2).

Information gleaned from re-referred patiens who have either failed to attend or dropped out, suggests that most of them are motivated to attend the clinic at least once in the hope of a miracle cure by medication. They rejected regular attendance for treatment for fear of the stigma attached to psychiatric treatment, often aggravated by the scorn of relatives.

Some are prevented by spouses, usually husbands, who feel that if talking is curative their own conversation should suffice, and it is not uncommon for a patient to say to the therapist, 'You are saying what my husband says', but it would seem to be more acceptable when said by the therapist.

Some reject any group method either through inability to integrate, fear of leakage of information, which might lead to loss of job, or fear of meeting 'lunatics' in the group.

Rejection of the therapist rarely occurs amongst neurotics, but commonly among those with disordered personalities. In a method where the therapist takes such an active part this is, in effect, rejection of the method. Among neurotics this probably leads to a few dropouts but usually to a request to join another class.

NOTES ON TABLE 3

Table 3 represents an attempt to ascertain whether it is justifiable to offer tutorial therapy to patients in all the categories shown. In some categories the numbers are too small to show more than a trend, if that, but it is nevertheless of interest that no significant differences at 5 per cent exist between the performance of the categories.

Dropout

This term is applied to patients who, so far as is known, were able to complete treatment but rejected the method.

Table 3 Comparison of factors which might give an indication of the suitability of the method to each category of patient

Category of neurotic patients	Dropout rates			Re-referral rates					Follow-up	
	Able to complete treatment	Dropouts		Completed treatment 1.4.76 to 31.3.77	Re-referred to the department up to 31.3.79				Followed up	Improvement assessed
					Totals		For further tutorial therapy			
	N	N	%	N	N	%	N	%	N	M%
(1) With no added complications	50	5	10	42	5	12	2	5	40	62
(2) Ditto, lightly affected	8	0	0	9	0	0	0	0	4	52
(3) Unlikely to integrate in a group	9	6	66	3	1	25	0	0	3	38
(4) With concurrent organic disease	5	0	0	5	1	20	0	0	3	52
(5) With personality disorder	11	7	64	2	1	50	0	0	0	
(6) With alcoholism	14	7	50	11	1	9	1	9	12	
(7) With concurrent endogenous depression in remission	14	3	21	9	4	44	1	11	6	42
Totals	111	28	25	81	13	16	4	5	68	57

Alcoholics were assessed at follow-up only on whether or not they were 'dry'; of the twelve followed up nine were dry a year after discharge and seven were dry 2 years after discharge from treatment.

No significant difference at 5 per cent were found to exist between the performances of the individual categories as regards dropout rates, re-referral rates or percentage improvement assessed at follow-up.

Re-referral

The patients enumerated were almost all re-referred only to this department; the figures given resulted from a search of the records on 1.4.79. Referral to other psychiatric departments without request for the records from this department is rare but can occur. Thus the figures are not to the standard of accuracy which would be required for a controlled study, but are of interest for comparing the performances of different categories of patients.

The period during which re-referral would have been noted was a minimum of 2 years, a maximum of 3 years and a mean of 31 months.

The differentiation between the total numbers re-referred and those of patients in need of further psychotherapy is of some interest. Of the five re-referrals in category (1) three only sought one conversation with a psychotherapist at a time of special stress. Of the other two, one had sought discharge before she was ready, discovered her error and returned for further treatment within a few weeks; the other had for her own convenience knowingly sought discharge before she was ready, and returned relying on the promise of a welcome which is extended to all discharged patients. Of the eight re-referrals in other categories one was seen twice at a time of special stress, one appears on Table 6 as a total failure of the method, one was not physically fit to withstand the stresses of the method, three with concurrent endogenous depression were re-referred for this condition while a fourth required further psychotherapy, and one alcoholic whose husband was drinking heavily, though *she* was still dry, sought support in tutorials for fear that she should relapse.

Follow-up

At the end of the year under review I was fortunate to find members of staff available to visit and perform a simple assessment of patients discharged from treatment during that year. These were two grade 6 community nurses, both experienced psychiatric nurses; neither had attended tutorial therapy nor taken any special interest in the method, in fact both were somewhat sceptical about the method when they undertook the follow-up. They visited each patient a year or more after completion of treatment, wrote a report on the patient's condition and made an assessment of the percentage improvement that could be attributed to the treatment. The excellence of the reports shows that trouble was taken and commonsense and understanding were applied.

In the absence of controls, follow-up assessments, even those of the before-and-after questionnaire type, are of very limited value. This informal follow-up is of interest in comparing the performance of patients in the different categories of whom the assessors had no knowledge.

It will be seen that, though no significant differences exist, categories (1), (2) and (4) show more favourable mean figures than categories (3),

(5), (6) and (7). Categories (1), (2) and (4) include only patients with no known added psychiatric complications, while categories (3), (5), (6) and (7) are composed of patients with added psychiatric complications. Comparison of these two groups is shown in Table 4.

Table 4 Comparison of the performances of neurotic patients with no added psychiatric complications as opposed to those with added psychiatric complications

Categories of neurotic patients	Dropout rates			Re-referral rates			Follow-up	
	Able to complete treatment	Dropouts		Completed treatment 1.4.76 to 31.3.77	Re-referred to the department 1.4.77 to 31.3.79		Followed up	Assessed improvement
	N	N	%	N	N	%	N	M%
With no added psychiatric complications (1), (2) and (4)	63	5*	8	56	6	11	47	60
With added psychiatric complications (3), (5), (6) and (7)	48	23*	48	25	7	28	9	41
Totals	111	28	25	81	13	16	56	57

*indicates significant difference at 5 per cent

NOTES ON TABLE 4

Between the performance of these two groups of patients the only significant difference at 5 per cent is in the dropout rate, which is significantly lower among those with no added psychiatric complications. The difference in re-referrals was not found to be quite significant at 5 per cent.

Among those with added psychiatric complications only patients in categories (3) and (7) were assessed for percentage improvement. (The two who completed treatment in category (5) were not traced, while the twelve in category (6) were assessed as being either 'dry' or not.) The assessed improvement for categories (1), (2) and (4) was compared with those for categories (3) and (7), even though the mean improvement differed by almost 20 per cent between these two groups, the result was not quite significant at the 5 per cent level.

Significance

Age of dropouts: In Table 2 significant difference at 5 per cent was found between the age of dropouts and the age of those who completed treatment in category (1) only. There were only five dropouts in category (1) so this may be a chance finding, but in fact it confirms a clinical impression with regard to category (1). In some other categories reasons for dropping out are essentially unrelated to age.

Dropout rates: In Table 4 significant difference at 5 per cent was found between the dropout rate of those with and without added psychiatric complications. Proportions dropping out were 0.48 of those with such complications, and 0.08 of those without. This result confirms expectations, if one takes the categories of those with added psychiatric complications:

Category (3), unlikely to integrate in a group. The description speaks for itself, but three out of nine completed treatment.

Categories, (5) with personality disorder, (7) with concurrent endogenous depression in remission. Psychotherapy will not alter personality nor cure psychosis, so it was only in the neurotic component of his whole problem that the patient could hope to benefit. Differentiation between two psychiatric components is more difficult for a patient than is differentiation between neurosis and physical disability or discomfort, though that too can be difficult. Moreover those who had previously been treated for psychosis had been conditioned to expect beneficial medicinal treatment for psychiatric conditions. Thus rejection of psychotherapy among patients in these two categories was to be expected and, perhaps, was sometimes well judged. In category (5) four out of eleven completed treatment, in category (7) eleven out of fourteen completed treatment.

(6) With alcoholism. The relapse rate in alcoholism is tragically high and nearly always accounts for dropouts in this category. Seven out of fourteen completed treatment.

In summary, 21 patients with added psychiatric complications completed treatment.

It appears likely that the policy of offering the treatment to all who *might* benefit and leaving them to select themselves operates at least as satisfactorily as would a psychiatrist's attempt to select. If that is so it would lead to economic use of the psychotherapeutic service because most patients who are unlikely to benefit will dropout. The reverse, however, does not apply, some dropouts are capable of benefiting and subsequently return. Whenever possible, dropouts should be seen again in clinic for consideration of other treatment, including individual psychotherapy, but not all are willing to attend.

Re-referral rates and assessed improvement: In Table 4 the almost significant differences in these factors support the expectation that those without added psychiatric complications are likely to derive greater benefit from psychotherapy than those with added psychiatric complications.

Conclusion: None of the results offers a reason to suggest that the opportunity to attend tutorial therapy should be withheld from patients in any of the categories.

Table 5   Factors which might be expected to influence performance. This table includes only patients in category (1) – those with no added complications, organic or psychiatric. It compares performances of those with and those without each of three factors

Category (1)	Completed treatment	Attend- ances	Re-referrals	Follow-up	
Patients having no added complications, organic				Followed up	Improvement
or psychiatric	N	M	%	N	M%
Totals of category (1)	70	25	10	40	62
Previously treated for neurosis by other methods	25	30	8	13	64
Not previously treated for neurosis by other methods	45	23	11	27	60
With problems of distance and transport	13	18	0	10	58
Without problems of distance and transport	57	27	12	30	63
With marital problems of some severity	14	34	7	6	63
Without marital problems	·56	23	11	34	61

No significant differences were found in any of the three sub-tables either in re-referral rate or percentage improvement

NOTES ON TABLE 5

Previously treated for neurosis by other methods

This description includes treatment for neurosis by psychotherapy in psychiatric departments, with or without the use of abreactants. It includes, in one case, 3 years' private treatment by psychoanalysis from which the patient said he had benefited though incompletely. It does not include medication and support given by general practitioners. In this year none who had previously been treated by behaviourist methods was referred.

Patients are included if they had been previously treated as described. Some had remitted under previous treatment. Three said they had benefited under previous treatment which they had been unable to complete.

With problems of distance and transport

Patients are so defined if they were resident 10 or more miles (16 km) from the hospital and/or in an area not served by public transport after 9 p.m., when tutorial classes end. Such patients were dependent on private transport or had to spend from about 5.30 p.m. to 10.30 p.m. away from home; in either case expense was considerable. Moreover, there were sometimes hazards for women travelling alone on public transport at night, particularly at pub-emptying time, walking through quiet residential streets while husbands, babysitting at home, could not meet them. Patients hardly needed to be agoraphobic in order to become anxious in this situation.

With marital problems of some severity

Patients are so defined if, at the time of presenting for treatment, they described marital discord ranging from battery to total, or near total, loss of interest, social and sexual, in the patient by the spouse, with or without unfaithfulness known to the patient. Four men and ten women are included. Patients who, at the time of presenting for treatment, were widowed or separated from their spouses are not included.

No significant differences were found in re-referral rates or assessed improvement in relation to any of the three factors. So far as small numbers permit, it may be deduced that these factors do not influence benefit from the treatment.

It is of some interest that the means of attendances are as might be expected in relation to the three factors. The mean attendances for category (1) patients as a whole were 25, but for those previously treated for neurosis by other methods the mean was 30 attendances. Over the years I have come to expect the patient who has received any other kind of psychotherapy to be a 'slow starter' in tutorials; he appears to need more time than others to adjust to the idea that he has to do it himself. Perhaps, if previous methods have failed, he is less trusting, so less inclined to accept the teaching and instructions and, of course, those who have proved resistant to one treatment may prove so to any treatment. However, I have noticed that those who have received long courses of neoanalytical psychotherapy, without improvement, tend to be intensely aware of and concerned with their 'feelings'. Persuading them to recognize some feelings, those of inferiority, for example, as false, and to try to use logic to abolish these emotional conditioned reflexes, can be time-consuming, because spending time with a doctor describing 'feelings' appears to have become part of a lifestyle.

Those with problems of distance and transport showed a mean of eighteen attendances, and the tendency to seek discharge as soon as possible was to be expected. Those with marital problems of some severity showed a mean of 34 attendances; it is noticeable that such patients often feel a need for the continued support of a friendly environment.

Table 6   Failure. This table gives some details of three patients who were treated during the year and did not respond to the method at all

Diagnosis	Category description	Category number	Sex	Age (years)	Attendances N
Compulsive eating	Unlikely to integrate	(3)	F	50	37
Anorexia nervosa	No added complications	(1)	F	22	19
Anxiety neurosis	No added complications	(1)	F	47	28

NOTES ON TABLE 6

The common factor amongst these three patients is that they attend under duress and, so far as is known, are the only patients to have attended under duress during the year. In the absence of pressure it is most probable that they would have dropped out. None of them integrated with the tutorial classes.

The first two were under pressure from husbands and relatives to obtain treatment. The first sought discharge when her weight had fallen from over 20 stone to 15 stone, but it is probable that she always exceeded her diet even as an inpatient. On regaining 20 stone she was re-referred, and then referred to a dental surgeon for wiring of teeth. Her assessed improvement at follow-up was 0 per cent. The second patient, a young woman at obvious risk of her life, from anorexia nervosa, was referred to a teaching unit when it became apparent that she would not respond to tutorial therapy. The report on discharge from that unit was not encouraging. Having been transferred at my wish she is listed as having been unable to complete treatment.

The third patient had been taking tranquillisers for many years, and had been previously treated for neurosis at another unit. She did not wish for treatment being content to take tranquillisers for life but, when her doctor retired, his replacement referred her for psychotherapy and withdrew the medication. She felt deeply aggrieved and insisted that she was in no need of treatment other than tranquillisers and, at follow-up, was awarded 1 per cent improvement.

It might be pleasant to assume complacently that these three patients were hopeless cases; but an ideal method of psychotherapy operated by ideal therapists would have found some means of overcoming their resistances; unlike dropouts they at least gave us time to do so.

Partial failure

Deductions can be made concerning partial failure by considering those patients in category (1) – with no added complications – who were followed up and assessed for percentage improvement a year or more after completing treatment. There were 40 such patients, one of whom is included under 'Failure' above (Table 6), leaving 39. These figures for percentage improvement are presented as if they were examination marks; the reader is left to decide the 'pass mark', thus neutralizing any objections concerning possible overestimations of improvement.

Spontaneous recovery

A patient who gives a history of 30 years of neurotic symptoms can hardly be judged to have made a spontaneous recovery if recovery

Table 7   Scale of assessed improvement of patients in category (1) – those with no added complications, organic or psychiatric

The number assessed as having improved	
0 to 9 per cent was	1 patient
10 to 19 per cent was	2 patients
20 to 29 per cent was	2 patients
30 to 39 per cent was	1 patient
40 to 49 per cent was	2 patients
50 to 59 per cent was	5 patients
60 to 69 per cent was	10 patients
70 to 79 per cent was	6 patients
80 to 89 per cent was	5 patients
90 to 99 per cent was	5 patients
Total	39

occurs under treatment, unlike one who gives a history of symptoms of brief duration. However, under treatment and at follow-up, a very different picture often emerges and it becomes evident that the symptoms of brief duration represented a volcanic eruption, matter driven up from inside by a lifelong pattern of maladjustment. If that pattern is not treated, though the existing acute symptoms may subside they will be likely to recur and, more important, the maladjustment will continue to bedevil the patient's life and that of his family.

Undoubtedly there are patients who enjoy an early remission of symptoms and discontinue treatment having gained very little from their attendance, but to identify and enumerate them with any reliability would be difficult if not impossible.

Re-reading records and follow-up reports on patients included in this review I am struck by the number who gave histories of symptoms of brief duration when first seen and, at follow-up a year or more after discharge from treatment, gave vivid descriptions of improvement in the quality of life. This, surely, is the purpose of psychotherapy? It does not matter that a few attend for treatment briefly and purposelessly; but it matters very much that treatment should be available to *all* who seek it and that it should be directed towards neurotic patterns of thought, reaction and attitude.

I offer one example, the first in the file that fulfils the requirements – symptoms of brief duration and treatment followed by improvement in the quality of life.

Miss YX, aged 23, single

Complained of: Overdose, depression, fed up with people, stopped speaking to people. One night boyfriend abandoned her by saying he had found someone else, she went home, took an overdose, was treated in casualty and admitted to hospital.

Six months previously: Felt giddy as though drunk, had frequent temper tantrums, saw her general practitioner and obtained medication, improved and discontinued medication but continued to have rows with everyone.

Childhood: Father strict, patient frightened of him. Mother spoilt her, always got her own way if she threw a tantrum. At other times mother threw things at the children. Patient was father's pet, ? mother jealous.

School and *work* records uneventful.

Sex: A bit short on boyfriends, gets fed up with them and leaves them; one or two have dropped her.

Diagnosis: Neurotic depression, immaturity, somewhat spoilt child.

Treatment: 26 attendances at tutorial therapy.

Follow-up: 21 months after completion of treatment.

Report by community nurse: Appetite very good, always hungry but doesn't eat to offset anxiety.

Sleep, drops off easily, wakes refreshed.

Employment, full-time, likes the job.

Relationships with colleagues – very good
Relationships with friends – plenty, no problems
Relationship with mother – made it up, now friends
Relationships with siblings – greatly improved.

Any psychiatric treatment since discharge? Psychiatrist – none, GP – none, no medication.

Did you benefit from group psychotherapy? Yes, I now take everything in its stride. I no longer explode when things don't go my way. I have grown up quite a bit. I try to use what Doctor taught me and if I do get tense I use the relaxation tape to calm me down and relax me.
How do you feel generally? Happy and gay. I don't worry any more. I am much more mature. I have a new boyfriend, we are saving up to get married soon. I have a flat of my own and this gives me confidence and independence.

Comment by community nurse: I found her to be confident, eager to answer questions and help in any way. From what she says it seems that treatment has given her insight into her previous behaviour so she can deal constructively with problems as they arise. She no longer 'demonstrates' when she cannot get her own way and uses what she has been taught effectively. She said, 'I am very happy and pleased with my life now'. Assessed percentage improvement 76 per cent.

This young woman, on the brink of marriage, had learnt to tolerate frustration and keep her temper. Thus a behaviour pattern learnt in early childhood had changed. In the interests of her unborn children this alone justified her treatment.

It is most probable that the acute symptoms of neurotic depression, which led to an overdose, would have subsided at the advent of a new boyfriend. It is possible that the behaviour pattern would have changed spontaneously within 3 years, but somewhat improbable as neither of her parents' similar immature behaviour patterns had changed before the time at which they reared their children. Thus it is most likely that, in this case, the chain of events leading to the neuroses of the parents being visited on the children unto the third and fourth generation has been broken as a result of treatment. Even if we discount the findings of the controlled study on the method (appendices (a) and (b)) and even if the treatment of as many as half our patients is judged to be purposeless, changes in the behaviour patterns of the other half, of which Miss YX is a fair sample, amply justify the time, effort and money expended, which per patient is not very great (see Table 8).

NOTES ON TABLE 8

Readers will appreciate that times given as having been spent on individual psychotherapy and administration are estimated, though as accurately as possible. Note that no allowance has been made for travelling time; this is impossible to estimate meaningfully because the distances travelled may vary greatly – in the cases of our therapists, travelling time varies from 2 or 3 minutes in one case, to an hour each way in another. Time spent on individual psychotherapy has, in my case, often been combined with travelling time, and the monthly 45 minutes spent sorting out the roll-books for each tutorial class and dictating letters to family doctors has invariably been found when a patient has failed to keep an appointment.

Table 8 Therapist's time expended per patient treated

Consultant for history and assessment	45 minutes
Tutorial classes, duration $\dfrac{2 \text{ hours}}{\text{mean attendance 7 patients}} = 17$ mins/patient/class	
mean attendances/patient 25 × 17 minutes =	7 hours 18 minutes
Individual psychotherapy for those few that need it	
3 patients × 3 sessions of 45 minutes = 405 minutes/year	
9 patients × 1 sessions of 45 minutes = 405 minutes/year	
Total 810 minutes/year	
Total patients discharged in year 81	
Estimated allowance per patient discharged	10 minutes
Therapist's time/patient expended in treatment, say	8 hours 15 minutes
Administration	
Consultant in clinic 45 minutes/month = 540 minutes/year	
Post-tutorial therapists' meetings	
a doctor 20 minutes/week	
2 therapists @ 20 minutes/week	
Total 60 minutes/week × 50 = 3000 minutes/year	
Total 3540 minutes/year	
Total patients discharged in year = 81 patients	
Estimated allowance per patient discharged $\dfrac{3540}{81}$ minutes =	45 minutes
Grand total	9 hours

The post-tutorial meetings are very informal; if a therapist has nothing to report or discuss he may leave immediately his tutorial class ends at 9 p.m. Generally two or three therapists, including at least one doctor, usually myself, will have matters to discuss which keep them for from 10 minutes to half an hour longer. When we have observers present, studying the method, all therapists who can stay will do so for anything up to an hour, but that is time spent teaching or learning as opposed to treating or administering.

SUMMARY OF THE AVERAGE COURSE OF TREATMENT AND PROGNOSIS

Calculated from the facts and figures given, a neurotic patient with no added complications, referred routinely, would be attending for treatment within less than a month from referral, while one referred as an emergency should attend his first tutorial within less than a week.

At the time of starting he would have a four-to-one chance of completing treatment which, on average, he would do after attending 25 tutorials over a period of 9 months.

After completing treatment his chance of seeking a further course of the treatment during the ensuing 2 to 3 years would be 1 in 20, while his chance of seeking a single appointment in the department would be 1 in 17.

13

A Review of Some Literature

A few quotations from Adler (1929) indicates the debt which this theory and method of psychotherapy owes to him:

> Every marked attitude of man can be traced back to an origin in childhood. . . . The child possesses a feeling of inferiority in its relations both to parents and the world. . . . The longer and more definitely the child feels his insecurity, the more he suffers from physical or marked mental weakness, the higher will this goal (of compensatory superiority) be placed and the more faithfully will it be adhered to.

With regard to the precipitating factor of a neurotic reaction he says, 'A single or repeated failure along the main line of human endeavour. This is the actual cause for the appearance of neurotic disease.' With regard to treatment he says, 'If the patient has gone to pieces under the pressure of reality the physician can *teach* him to come to terms with both reality and society' (my italics).

Pavlov (1926) established beyond doubt the importance of training in the aetiology of neurosis, and demonstrated the mechanism through which it occurs, for which he coined the term 'conditioned reflex'. Through the application of conditioned reflexes to which they had been trained he caused neurotic reactions in dogs. In the absence of training the neuroses could not have been caused. From this it may be deduced that the inevitably complex training applied to civilized man in infancy and childhood offers ample opportunity for the seeds of neurosis to be sown.

All Pavlov's dogs, however stable their personalities, reacted neurotically when sufficient strain was applied. Thus we cannot assume that the primary cause of neurotic illness is a congenital personality *fault*, an assumption which is sometimes given as a reason for offering only supportive as opposed to active treatment. Dejerine (Dejerine and Gaukler, 1911) says of the neurotic that he takes life too seriously and is often too scrupulous and too loyal. This supports my belief in the neurotic's high congenital loading of goodwill, but it can hardly be described as a fault.

Wolpe (1958) described the application of the learning theory and desensitization in the treatment of neurosis, using the techniques of relaxation, assertion and approach to the feared object or situation. Eysenck (1960) described a theory of the aetiology of neurosis in terms of the learning theory.

Dejerine and Gaukler (1911), Dubois (1913) and Lewis (1956) advocate explaining to the patient the reasons for his condition.

Schilder (1936) recommends that a group therapist should take an active part in treatment. Pratt (1945) used a lecture method for treating groups of twenty neurotic patients. Slavson (1947) describes a method of managing a group similar to the one I have described.

Lewis (1956) says it is important, '. . . to understand the development of the patient's illness. . . in terms of real experience rather than hypothetical forces'. Rogers (1942) says, '. . . this understanding of the self and acceptance of the self is the next important aspect of the whole process'; and, 'It is the courage to face life and the obstacles which it presents which is the aim of therapy'.

Hobson (1974), describing the needs of the patient, writes, '. . . giving and receiving, a sharing with another person who opens himself to her and is not only 'playing a part' (although that part might be necessary sometimes). She asks for a genuine conversation in mutual trust which can free her to *explore* not only alone but also together with another person.' Bromberg (1961) says, '. . . the therapeutic staff is not unwilling to expose, to a limited degree, their own anxieties and tensions'. Wolpe (1958) says of the patient, 'He is given the feeling that the therapist is unreservedly on his side'.

Atkin (1959) condemns the use of tranquillisers for the treatment of neurosis as being a quick way of assuaging the symptoms instead of trying to cure the illness.

Slavson (1947), Johnson (1963), Wolf and Swartz (1962) all advise the exclusion of psychotic and psychopathic patients from groups intended for the treatment of neurosis.

I chose these brief quotations and descriptions from a shortlist of authors because they support different aspects of the theory and method which I have described.

It was in July 1981 when, having practised the method for nearly twenty years and published a paper entitled, 'Teaching neurotic patients to treat themselves' (Bovill, 1973) that I found support for this, one of the central themes of the method. Professor Marks (1981) writes advising psychiatrists to teach neurotic patients to treat themselves by behaviourist methods. He points out that this is not unduly time-consuming and that it can be practised individually or in groups. It is very satisfactory to now find myself supported on these points by such an authority.

He also makes a point which I thought of special interest in a general sense. He says, 'Behavioural psychotherapy has systematized many principles which have been used in common sense fashion for centuries'. Sensible people have doubtless been using these principles for training children and animals since the dawn of history. They are a matter of common knowledge to stockmen and dog-trainers throughout the world. Of course this does not belittle the honour due to Pavlov and his successors who proved the importance of these principles in the aetiology and treatment of neurosis.

Appendix (a)

A TRIAL OF GROUP PSYCHOTHERAPY FOR NEUROTICS* †

In peripheral hospitals and their crowded outpatient clinics many neurotics are treated, sometimes for a number of years, with sedatives or tranquillizers, a few words of sympathy and encouragement and, often electroplexy. The reasons often given for failure to offer psychotherapy are that it is of doubtful benefit or that it is too time-consuming.

This study was carried out in a peripheral hospital, St. Crispin, Northampton, by myself, then a senior registrar, while working as ward doctor on an acute admission ward. It was designed to compare the efficacy of the routine methods of treating neurotics against a consistent course of group psychotherapy and relaxation. The comparison was made primarily in terms of re-admission rate: but also in terms of doctors' time expended on the two methods. The results have been reported in detail, together with a discussion of the literature (Bovill, 1965), in a thesis for the degree of M.D. This is available at the Library of the University of London, at the Institute of Psychiatry, London, at the Westminster Hospital, and at St. Andrew's Hospital and St. Crispin Hospital, both of Northampton.

Conduct of the trial

The trial was conducted over 37 months, patients were collected in

*First published in *British Journal of Psychiatry* (1972), **102**, 285–92. Reproduced by kind permission of the Editor.
† The subject of a thesis for a degree of MD, London, 1965.

hospital during the first 13 months, and studied from the time of leaving hospital till the end of the 37 months, except in the cases of three patients who were lost to sight before this. The mean period in study was 30 months, the range was 17 to 37 months. Table A.1, describing the clinical material handled during the this time, shows how it was that out of 72 patients seen at group sessions only 36 fulfilled the requirements of the trial.

Table A.1   Classification of patients seen at group sessions during the 37 months of collection and study of the compared series

	Years			Total
	1	2	3	
Treated neurotics, hospitalized	36	23	30	89
Treated neurotics, non-hospitalized	8	13	9	30
Treatment refusers	3	0	4	7
Rediagnosed psychotic	19	14	13	46
Addicts and alcoholics	3	6	2	11
Disruptive psychopaths	1	1	0	2
Miscellaneous others	2	1	4	7
Short hospitalizations	0	7	5	12
Aged under 18	0	0	4	4
Not available for follow-up	0	7	1	8
	72	72	72	216

Treated patients were collected from those in my care, while controls were collected from those in the care of senior colleagues. Random selection being impracticable, a method of accepting all comers was substituted, all patients who fell within specified requirements being included.

Requirements for inclusion were: sex female, ages 18 to 59, intelligence within the normal range, physical condition at least adequate to allow a housewife to carry out her work, and absence of evidence of psychosis, epilepsy, addiction or reaction to severe but transient circumstances. At least one day of a course of hospitalization was required to fall within the first 13 months of the study period.

The course of hospitalization leading to collection for the series was required to be reasonably unexceptional. Three Treated and 1 Control patients were rejected because all or nearly all their time in hospital had occurred during their doctors' leaves. One Control was rejected because she left hospital against advice, and 3 more Controls were rejected because they remained in hospital for more than 6 months which, it was thought, suggested exceptional chronicity and dependance. The course of hospitalization leading to acceptance for the series was ordinarily required to last at least 10 days to give time for assessment and to suggest a measure of co-operation: but 2 Treated patients were accepted after short inpatient treatment, both were fully co-operative but left to attend to genuine family emergencies.

Nine Controls with severe social problems which could not be matched amongst the Treated were rejected, the intention being to bias results, if at all, against the Treated. The performance of these 9 proved that the bias occurred as intended. Treated patients with problems which could not be matched amongst the Controls were not rejected.

A requirement which applied only to the Treated was that patients should not disrupt group sessions unduly; only one, a young psychopath, was rejected from the series for this reason (and was later transferred to Rampton though not by me). Two others proved too disruptive for sessions, but these were subsequently rediagnosed as schizophrenic.

A follow-up of at least a year was obviously essential, and in this Treated patients were found to be more co-operative than Controls; 7 Controls could not be traced at the end of the first year and were rejected for this reason. Thereafter no Controls were lost to sight except one who died of natural causes: but 2 Treated patients, who were studied for 17 and 30 months respectively, were lost to sight before the end of the study. These three are included in the study.

In the age group 50 to 59 there were patients potentially available for both groups who were excluded for doubtful diagnosis; in this age group endogenous depression often presents with an exacerbation of neurotic symptoms which have been of minor significance throughout life, the patient may respond to hospitalization and medication and leave hospital before a firm diagnosis has been made. And, with regard to the Treated, as the stigma of psychiatric hospitalization still bears hardly on this age group and was found to lead to resistance to attendance at group sessions, it was not thought justifiable to apply pressure in the presence of a doubtful diagnosis.

Apart from these exceptions all those who fell within the specifications were included.

Treated patients were potentially collected for inclusion in the trial on attending the first group session after admission to hospital; this often occurred before a firm diagnosis had been reached, so some rejections for diagnostic reasons occurred subsequently. Controls were collected from their case sheets after discharge from hospital; this, of course, ensured the blind treatment of Controls. All patients who, at any time during the trial, were firmly rediagnosed as psychotic were then rejected; in cases of doubt independent confirmation was sought.

In order to confirm the diagnoses of all patients in the study and thus confirm the diagnostic parity of the two groups, and in order to obtain uniformity of diagnostic labels used throughout both groups, the case sheets of all patients were reviewed by an independent consultant psychiatrist. The diagnostic labels which he attached are those used in this paper.

The criterion for success was the patient's capacity to remain at home, so periods of rehospitalization for both groups were tabulated and compared. It was thought that results thus claimed required confirmation in terms of patient well-being. Simple questionnaire forms were prepared for application to patients and relatives; these requested information on symptoms complained of on admission – were these better, the same or worse; on behaviour, such as the ability to go out alone and to work; and on general demeanour. Questionnaires were also prepared for the family doctors; these were designed to assess the amount of attention and medication the patient was requiring and the opinion of the doctor on her condition. These questionnaires were completed during a few weeks following the end of the trial; those for the doctors were posted, while those for the patients and relatives were filled in by social workers visiting patients in their homes. Scoring of questionnaires was by an independent doctor.

Treatment methods

All patients on reaching hospital saw their doctors for the usual initial interview for history, assessment and diagnosis, and all received medication as seemed advisable.

Treatment of controls. Controls were treated by the routine methods in current use; these included individual interviews with the doctor of a psychotherapeutic nature, and some were referred to outpatient clinics on leaving hospital, but it is perhaps significant that these outpatients were rarely treated by the doctor who they knew in hospital.

Just over two-thirds of the Controls received electroplexy, a mean of 7.2 convulsions per patient treated was given. This treatment was thought by some doctors to be useful therapy in some cases of neurotic depressive reaction, anxiety reaction, hysterical reaction and inadequate personality.

Treatment of treated patients. Treated patients were usually included in group psychotherapy sessions within 4 days of reaching hospital; they were then dependent on these for psychotherapy; but they saw the doctor individually weekly, briefly, for administration and adjustment of medication. They attended two group sessions a week while in hospital and usually one a week after leaving hospital for as long as they wished to attend; when they decided to discontinue attendance they were invited to attend again at any time without formality. Outpatients wishing to see the doctor alone could do so after a group session, but they were discouraged from discussing then matters which could have been brought up in the group, and in fact they rarely attempted to do so.

Each group session lasted two hours, and the mean number of patients attending was 10. Three group sessions were held each week; two held in the hospital accepted in- and outpatients, one held 25 miles away was for outpatients in that area. The groups were open, 72 patients were introduced to them during the first 13 months, of whom 39 fulfilled the requirements of the trial (3 dropouts), and a further 72 were introduced to them during each of the two succeeding years (see Table A.1). The 36 included in the study were thus no favoured few.

Relaxation classes were attended four times a week in hospital, and once, in conjunction with a group session, after leaving hospital. The method was after Garmany (1952); classes were conducted by the remedial gymnast, Mr. R. Billingham.

Three patients were sent into hospital by consultants for electroplexy; a mean of six convulsions per patient were given. Having shown no improvement these patients were then treated with group psychotherapy. The time these three spent in hospital for electroplexy prior to receiving psychotherapy is included in the mean time hospitalized in the initial hospitalization (Table A.2), which might thus be reduced from 39 days to 37 days/patient. This extra time spent in hospital also enters into the calculation of mean doctor hours expended per patient (Table A.2).

Doctors' time. Detailed estimates were made of the expenditure of doctors' time on the Treated and Control groups. These were, of necessity, rough estimates but they are thought to be realistic. These show that the time expended per patient is almost equal for the two

Table A.2   Features of treatment and management (±
= estimated figures)

	Treated	Controls
Number in series	36	36
Mean days in hospital in the initial hospitalization	38.9	40.75*
Electroplexy, number of patients treated	3	25
Mean Dr.-Pt. psychotherapeutic sessions per patient:		
Individual inpatient ±	2	6.8
Outpatient clinic		5.6
Group inpatient	8.9	
Group outpatient	22.2	
Totals	33.1	12.4
Percentage treated as outpatients	94%	66%
Mean patient hours spent with doctor (± controls)	79.7	11.4
Mean doctor hours expended per patient, ±	11.1	11.4
Mean relaxation class attendances per patient	17.33	

*Indicates no statistically significant difference between
the two groups at 5 per cent.

methods of treatment. In the short term the conventional method
applied to the Controls was the more economical of time; but the readmission to hospital of Controls was so much heavier than that of the
Treated that over 37 months of the trial period the time expended on
both groups became equal. It is of note that, for the same expenditure
of doctors' time, the Treated patients averaged 80 hours in a psychotherapeutic situation against a maximum of 11½ hours for the
Controls. This, of course, is attributable to the group method.

Comparative data for Treated and Control groups are shown in
Table A.3. The fact that each group contains the same number of
patients, 36, was accidental. There was no psychologist attached to the
hospital, but psychological tests were arranged when this proved
possible, though some patients failed to attend for them; no statistical
difference at 5 per cent was found between the performance in the trial
of tested and untested patients. The previous admissions of one
Treated patient were excluded from the Table in order to obtain a
realistic mean, she having been previously hospitalized for 381 days.
Matching of the groups under marital status is not good: but
Malzberg's (1940) figures indicate that spinsters and feme-sole are

TUTORIAL THERAPY

Table A.3 Comparative data of the two groups of 36 patients

			Treated	Controls
Age		Mean	38.8	34.9*
I.Q. Raven Matrices	(N 27, 24)	,,	107.8	107.9*
V.Q. Mill Hill	(N 27, 24)	,,	94.3	92.2*
Neuroticism M.P.I.	(N 27, 24)	,,	35.2	31.1*
Extroversion M.P.I.	(N 27, 24)	,,	24.7	21.1*
Duration of history in years				
	(N 36, 36)	,,	8.2	8.3*
Days previously in hospital per				
patient	(N 36, 36)	,,	15.5	16.5*
	(N 35, 36)			
Patients previously hospitalized				
		Number	16	15*
		(36, 36)		
Marital status:				
Married and living with husband				
at start of study		,,	27	35
Spinsters throughout the study		,,	6	1
Feme-sole at start of study		,,	3	0
Separated during the study		,,	0	2
Widows at start of study		,,	0	0
Widowed during the study		,,	3	0
In social Class II		,,	4	3
III		,,	8	7
IV		,,	21	23
V		,,	3	3
Diagnosis (often multiple):				
Anxiety reaction		,,	24	26
Depressive reaction		,,	20	25
Hysterical reaction		,,	6	6
Phobic reaction		,,	9	8
Somatic symptoms		,,	12	8
Hypochondriacal reaction		,,	3	2
Pathological Personality:				
Inadequacy or passive ·				
dependence		,,	1	4
Antisocial or aggressive		,,	6	0
Social problems, patients with:		,,	24	20
Money troubles		,,	9	4
Marital problems, separations		,,	3	2
rearing children alone		,,	4	2
disharmony ± violence		,,	12	12
Unwilling, pregnancies,				
married		,,	2	0
spinsters		,,	2	0
Problem children		,,	5	4
Husband's ill health		,,	6	2
Bereavements within family				
household during or up to a				
year before study		,,	4	3
Living alone		,,	7	0
Language problem, of ·				
foreign birth		,,	1	0
Total of problems		,,	55	29

* Indicates no statistically significant difference at 5 per cent.

more likely to be hospitalized than married women or widows; and Parkes (1964) found that, for 18 months after bereavement, widows are likely to need medical support, so it would appear that this inequality in matching favoured the Controls. Social Class is after Hollingshead and Redlich (1958). Matching is poor amongst pathological personalities, but it will be seen in Table A.4 that omission of patients with these diagnoses does not materially alter the main result.

Results

Results are shown in Table A. 4. For reasons of family, distance and transport, 9 treated patients discontinued treatment before they felt ready to do so; a difference in the mean performances of these as opposed to the rest is detectable and is shown in Table A.4. At least one well-being assessment was obtained for 71 out of the 72 patients in the series, the exception, a Control, died during the trial.

Table A.4

		Treated	Controls
Number in series		36	36
Mean duration of study in months (Range 17 to 37)		29.0	29.2
Mean days rehospitalized per patient during study		3.1	22.7
Ditto for 'Fully Treated' patients numbering 27		2.7	
Ditto for 9 patients who discontinued treatment early		4.3	
Ditto adding 3 dropouts to 36 treated, total 39		3.5	
Ditto extracting ill-matched classes of patients:			
Pathological personalities, antisocial etc.		2.6	21.7
Pathological personalities, inadequate etc.		3.1	21.9
Number of patients rehospitalized		8	16
Number of rehospitalizations		10	22
Mean scores of well-being assessments:			
Family doctors	(N 36, 34)	30.9	19*
Patients	(N 32, 32)	82.8	76.6
Relatives	(N 28, 31)	82.7	77.4
Percentage improved, family doctors' estimates	(N 35, 34)	83	65

*Indicates differences statistically significant at 5 per cent.

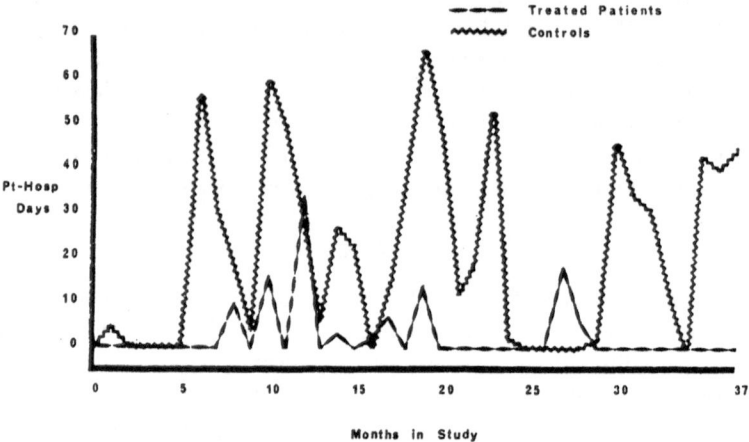

Figure A.1   Pattern of rehospitalization

Patterns of readmissions. Comparison of the pattern or distribution of readmissions of Treated and Controls is of interest, these are shown in Figure A.1. It will be seen that readmissions of Controls are distributed evenly throughout the period in study and might therefore be expected to continue thus indefinitely. But those of the Treated, with one exception, fade out at about the mid-point of the study period. This single readmission in the second half of the study period was one of the 9 patients mentioned above who, for reasons of distance, had failed to continue outpatient treatment for as long as she wished. It is of note that no Treated patient who had completed treatment was readmitted: readmissions occurred either during treatment or amongst those who had discontinued treatment before they wished to do so.

In order to study further the usefulness of the method of treatment, patients admitted in the following two years, who fulfilled the same requirements, were reviewed (see Table A.1). The results of this uncontrolled study are available in Bovill (1965); they show a similar performance with regard to rehospitalization.

Some further information about the Treated patients is of interest (Table A.4). The way in which these patients were accumulated and were discharged or left led to the attendance pattern of Figure A.2. Psychiatrists with preconceptions about the endlessness of psychotherapy may be relieved to see that in fact patients were being dis-

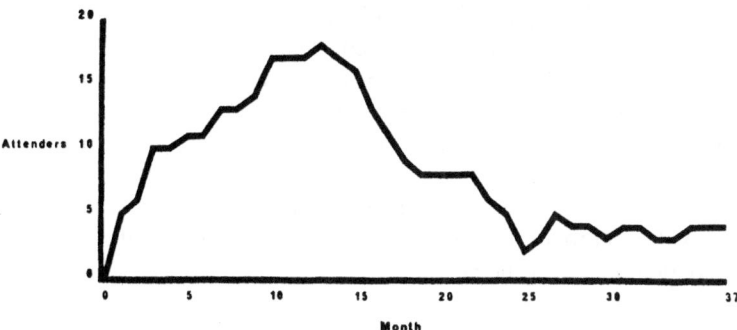

Figure A.2   Monthly pattern of attendances

charged throughout the study. But, of course, Figure A.2 does not reflect the total numbers present at group meetings; these were being continuously augmented by new admissions, and so remained approximately constant (Table A.1).

Table A.5   Duration of treatment and of independence of treated patients

Number of patients treated	36
Mean months in study	30
Mean months under treatment	8.8
Mean months without treatment	22.2
Mean months after final discharge and up to end of study	19.4
Patients who returned for further treatment after discharge	8 = 22%
Patients almost continuously under treatment	2 = 5.5%
Patients independent at end of study	30 = 83%

It will be seen that at the mid-point of the study patients attending had fallen to 8, and at the end of the study to 4; but shortly after the end of the study 2 more sought further help so that the number claimed as independent is 30, 83 per cent. It is interesting that the same percentage was estimated as being improved by the family doctors. Figure A.2 shows that in the 25th month attendance fell to 2; these 2 were continuously under treatment. Thereafter it fluctuated as patients returned for short periods of further treatment.

Factors which might influence prognosis. In considering factors which may be supposed to influence the amount of psychotherapy which patients might require, the 27 patients who continued treatment for as long as they wished were reviewed. The factors reviewed were: age (20–59), I.Q. (R.P.M. 72–130) and duration of symptoms (0–28) years. Individual scores for these factors were graphed against the number of sessions each patient elected to attend. No clear pattern emerged on any graph.

Thus, on the evidence of this small study, review of these factors is of no value in prognosticating the amount of group psychotherapy which a patient may feel she needs.

Discussion

Within its limits as to time and numbers the results of the trial suggest strongly that group psychotherapy and relaxation are beneficial to neurotics, and that a consistent course of this treatment can be provided without expending more doctor's time than would be expended on the routine methods. The importance of the group method was obviously crucial; it was responsible for the essential economy in doctors' time, for the flexibility which enabled patients to return to treatment when they felt the need, and for the fact that Treated patients spent a mean of 7 hours in a psychotherapeutic situation for every hour so spent by the Controls. But another factor which is thought to have been of great importance to the success of the treatment was the continuity of doctor, method and fellow patients through the point in time of leaving hospital; this continuity is not always obtained under peripheral N.H.S. conditions, because it is common for a junior doctor to care for the patient on the ward while a consultant undertakes aftercare in the outpatient clinic, and even where the ward doctor, senior or junior, takes outpatient clinics, it may be geographically unacceptable for a patient to attend his clinic. But my experience led me to suppose that this geographical unacceptability is often either an unjustifiable assumption or a doctor factor rather than a patient factor. I found most patients prepared to put themselves to very considerable trouble and expense to continue treatment under the doctor they had known in hospital.

Theory and method of psychotherapy. This was simple and didactic, it was designed to increase self respect and self understanding, to break up undesirable habits of thought, and thus to assist the patient to cope successfully with the difficulties of life. Each patient in turn introduced a subject for discussion, usually a symptom or problem, and this was discussed with me while the remaining patients acted as audience.

Interpatient discussion occurred, but did not form a large part of the proceedings. Emotional outbursts were almost unknown in sessions, but were often reported as having occurred elsewhere and were then discussed in sessions. This matter will not be discussed further, psychiatric literature being already satiated with accounts of psychotherapeutic theories and methods.

Dropouts. Dropouts were defined as patients who, while meeting the requirements of the trial, and having attended at least one group session, failed to attend ten sessions. Those who attended at least ten sessions were included in the trial.

Thirty-nine patients fulfilled the requirements for the trial and attended at least one group session, 3 patients failed to attend ten sessions and so were classified as dropouts. This is a dropout rate of 8 per cent, which contrasts remarkably with Brill's (1964) 43 per cent dropout rate: but there are differences between the two studies which may account for this.

Dropouts could only occur amongst the Treated, and so represented a possible source of bias between the two groups. This was overcome by including the figures for readmissions of dropouts amongst the results of the trial; they will be found in Table A.4.

Possible sources of bias. Anyone familiar with the work of a junior doctor in a peripheral hospital will know that I was never in a position to select patients for admission to my care or to that of any other doctor. From amongst those in my care I could have rejected for treatment those with a bad prognosis had I known of any reliable prognostic factors with which to guide my choice; but, though laboriously, my records and the hospital records room could provide proof that no suitable patient was rejected from either group of the series.

I was, of course, never in a position to influence the management of Controls: but it might be thought that I could have reduced, unjustifiably, the inpatient time of Treated patients. Had I done so I would have first risked suicidal attempts; 12 out of the 36 had previous attempts on record, none occurred during the trial. Secondly, the family doctor, following the usual procedure, would have requested readmission from the consultant concerned. This never occurred. The criterion for success, time spent rehospitalized, was the subject of a discovery in the 18th month of the trial. Previously I had intended to use well-being assessments only. Figure A.1 shows that by the 18th month the divergence between the hospitalizations of the two groups of patients was already well established.

Summary

A trial on the outcome of treatment was carried out on two groups of 36 initially hospitalized neurotic patients. The controls received individual psychotherapeutic sessions, some received electroplexy, and some were referred to outpatient clinics on leaving hospital; these were the routine methods in current use. The Treated patients joined open psychotherapeutic groups in hospital and continued attendance after leaving hospital for as long as they wished or could arrange to do so. They were also taught relaxation. The mean time in study was 30 months, the range was 17 to 37 months. The main criterion of success was the extent to which patients attained independence of the hospital as shown inversely by days spent rehospitalized during the trial, at the end of which results stood at 7:1 in favour of the Treated. Results of well-being assessments were also significantly favourable. Doctors' time expended on the two methods was found to be equal. Treated patients were under treatment by group psychotherapy and relaxation for a mean of nearly nine months, range 2–31; independent after final discharge for a mean of 19½ months, range 0–34; 83 per cent were regarded as being independent of treatment at the end of the trial. No relationship was found to exist between the number of sessions which treated patients elected to attend, and age, I.Q. or duration of symptoms. It was concluded that a consistent course of group psychotherapy and relaxation is beneficial to neurotic patients and that this is not uneconomical in doctors' time.

Acknowledgements

My grateful thanks are due to Professor Sir Aubrey Lewis, to Dr Andrew Graham and Dr Paul Rogers of St. Crispin Hospital, and to many members of that hospital's staff, especially Mr R. Billingham and Mr John Lawe. Also to Dr Letemendia of Littlemore Hospital, Dr Hunter of Coney Hill Hospital, Dr R. Kellner of Liverpool University, Professor A. E. Maxwell of the Institute of Psychiatry, University of London, Dr A. Barr of the Oxford Regional Hospital Board, and the late Miss P. Bennett of Broadmoor Hospital.

References

Bovill, D. (1965). 'Continuity of Psychotherapy in the Neuroses, A Compared Trial.' Thesis for the degree of M.D. London.

Brill, N. G. (1964). 'A comparative study of the effectiveness of psychotherapy.' Paper read at the 6th International Congress of Psychotherapy.

Garmany, G. (1952). *Muscle Relaxation as an Adjunct to Psychotherapy.* London: Actinic Press

Hollingshead, A. B. and Redlich, F. C. (1958). *Social Class and Mental Illness.* New York: John Wiley.

Malzberg, B. (1940). *Social and Biological Aspects of Mental Disease.* New York: State Hospital Press.

Parkes, C. H. (1964). 'Effects of bereavement on physical and mental health, a study of the medical records of widows.' *British Medical Journal,* ii, 274–9.

A synopsis of this paper was published in the December 1971 *Journal.*

Diana Bovill, M.D., M.R.C.Psych., D.P.M., *Consultant Psychiatrist, St. Andrew's Hospital, Northampton*

(*Received 30 September 1970*)

Appendix (b)

AN OUTCOME STUDY OF GROUP PSYCHOTHERAPY*

In 1975 a long-term follow-up was undertaken on patients collected as inpatients, treated and studied in 1962–64 (Bovill, 1972). Treatment was by didactic group psychotherapy and relaxation. Treatment was for a mean of six months and of 30 sessions, treatment remained available on demand for a mean of two years after discharge from attendance. In 1975 30 Treated patients and 24 Control patients were traced out of the original 36 in each group. The criterion of success was, as before, the inverse of days spent rehospitalized. The success ratio fell from 7 : 1 in 1962–64 to 2½ : 1 in 1965–74 and 2 : 1 in the single year 1974. This fall was expected in view of the known spontaneous recovery rate operating on the Controls.

Introduction

A study of group psychotherapy was undertaken at St. Crispin Hospital, Northampton, in 1961–64. This was the subject of a thesis (Bovill, 1965), and a paper (Bovill, 1972), of which the summary reads: 'A trial on the outcome of treatment was carried out on two groups of 36 recently admitted neurotic patients. The Controls received individual psychotherapeutic sessions, some received electroplexy and

*First published in *British Journal of Psychiatry* (1977), **131**, 95–8. Reproduced by kind permission of the Editor.

198

some were referred to outpatient clinics on leaving hospital. The Treated patients joined open psychotherapeutic groups in hospital and continued attendance after leaving hospital for as long as they wished or could arrange to do so. They were also taught relaxation.

'The study started for each patient at the time of leaving hospital. The mean time in study was 30 months, the range was 17 to 37 months. The main criterion of success was the extent to which patients attained independence of the hospital, as shown inversely by days spent rehospitalized during the study, at the end of which results stood at 7 : 1 in favour of the Treated. Results of well-being assessments were also favourable. Doctors' time expended on the two methods was found to be equal . . .'

In 1975 a long-term follow-up on the same population was undertaken. Thirty Treated patients and 24 Controls were traced and their readmissions to hospital between 1 January 1965 and 31 December 1974 recorded. The Treated then had a mean time in study of 12.3 years, the Controls of 12.0 years.

The patient population

Requirements for inclusion were age 18–59 years, IQ 70 + , and absence of gross organic disease (Table B.1).

Treatment

After the initial history-taking session, which included an introduction to psychotherapy, Treated patients were dependent on group sessions, being usually seen individually only for administrative purposes and adjustment of medication. Occasionally a patient would seek an individual session for the discussion of an especially private matter, but this was not common. The Controls were treated individually with psychotherapy of a counselling nature, analytically orientated. Medication was given to all patients as appropriate, but I am unwilling to discharge a patient from group attendance until all psychotropic medication has been withdrawn. I rarely give electroconvulsive therapy to neurotic patients, though I am not in general opposed to physical treatment. The two Treated patients who received electroconvulsions did so on the instruction of the consultant, I being a senior registrar at that time.

Treated patients were discharged from treatment at their own

Table B.1   The patient population in the study

Collection of patients for this study took place at the end of the first hospitalization occurring between 1 December 1961 and 31 December 1962; this is described as the 'Collection Hospitalization'

	Treated	Controls
Number of patients traced in 1975	30	24
At 'Collection Hospitalization' mean age (range 18–59 years)	39.6	33.2
Mean duration of symptoms in years	8.1	8.3
Percentage previously hospitalized	47%	33%
Mean days in hospital before 'Collection Hospitalization'	16.0	12.6
During 'Collection Hospitalization'	39.5	45.7
Before the start of this study	55.5	58.3

Table B.2   Treatment given between 1 December 1961 and 31 December 1964 to 30 Treated Patients and 24 Controls

	Treated		Controls	
	Number treated	Mean treatments per patient treated	Number treated	Mean treatments per patient treated
Doctor/patient therapeutic sessions				
Individual I.P. (estimation)	30	2.0	24	6.8
Group I.P. and O.P.	30	32.3		
Electroconvulsions	2	4.0	19	7.0
Relaxation classes	28	18.4		
Follow-up appointments attendances	28	21.0	17	10.4

Note: The follow-up appointments attendances of the Treated patients were at group sessions; those of the Controls were at out-patient clinics

Table B.3   Time spent by Treated patients under treatment and independent of treatment between 1 December 1961 and 31 December 1964

Number of patients treated	30
who returned for further treatment after initial discharge	7
continuously under treatment while it was available	1
Mean number of months in study	30
attending groups sessions	6
independent of treatment	24
after last attendance	20

Table B.4   Results in terms of time spent rehospitalized for 30 Treated patients and 24 Controls

| | 1962–64 | | 1965–74 | | 1962–74 | |
	Treated	Controls	Treated	Controls	Treated	Controls
Years in study, mean/patient	2.5	2.5	9.7	9.6	12.3	12.0
Percentage of patients readmitted	20%	42%	17%	37%	30%	58%
Days in hospital, mean/patient	3.0	21	10	27	13	48
Ratio	1:7		1:2½		1:3½	

request; they were not pressured to accept discharge but were advised that they were free to return to group attendance at any time; only seven did so but others telephoned to make sure that treatment was still available to them, which suggests that availability of treatment was a supporting factor. This support was deliberately withdrawn on 1 January 1965; thereafter patients in the study were dependent on the ordinary facilites provided by the hospital, with one exception, a patient who sought me out in my new appointment and there attended four group sessions in 1966.

Results

Those patients traced in 1975 number 30 Treated and 24 Controls, as opposed to 36 in each group on 31 December 1964, but the rehospitalization ratio of 7 : 1 for the first three years in study still holds good for this reduced number of patients, while figures for the numbers of readmitted and number of readmissions correspond almost equally well. This suggests that those traced are a representative sample of the whole, which lends support to the validity of the results for the subsequent ten years.

In round figures the expectations from the first 2½ years in study for the ensuing ten years would have been that the Treated would be readmitted for a mean of 12 days and the Controls for a mean of 84, but, in fact, while the Treated approximately fulfilled this expectation (10.4 days/patient) the performance of the Controls improved considerably (26.8 days/patient). Sloane et al. (1975) have published similar findings over a shorter period, and Wallace and White (1959) found a spontaneous recovery rate of 65 per cent in less than three years, so the improvement in performance of Controls in this study is not unexpected, but their performance has not equalled that of the Treated in 1974. In that year it stood at an approximate 2 : 1 for patients readmitted, readmissions and days hospitalized.

Availability of the treatment was discontinued on 1 January 1965; had it not been, the performance of the Treated would probably have continued to improve. No Treated patient was readmitted to hospital after her discharge from attendance at group sessions while the opportunity to return to them was still available to her.

I regret that in 1975 I was unable to obtain well-being scores, as I did in 1965 when the Mental Welfare Officers visited and filled in questionnaires for patients and relatives; 94 per cent of patients then traced agreed to co-operate with Mental Welfare Officers, whereas only 60 per cent of those traced in 1975 agreed to co-operate with Social Workers.

Discussion

The method of psychotherapy is based upon simple and direct instruction regarding the origins of neurotic symptoms and methods of managing them more appropriately. Behavioural techniques are recommended, together with exploration of interpersonal difficulties. Emphasis is placed on creating and maintaining a safe and encouraging group culture which facilitates the possibility of patients finding their own solutions to their difficulties. Some degree of therapist disclosure is shown, in order to reduce feelings of shame among the group members. A brief account has been published (Bovill, 1973). The intention in evolving this method was to provide treatment for the large numbers of neurotics who are referred to peripheral hospitals and to whom conventional methods are inapplicable because neither therapist's nor, in many cases, patients' time, is available in sufficient quantity.

With regard to numbers in 1962–64 72 patients/year were offered treatment, which was given in three group sessions/week; then, as now, inpatients attended twice weekly, outpatients once. In 1973 94 patients were offered treatment at four group sessions/week. In April 1976 66 patients were on the rolls for weekly attendance, 8 of whom were attending twice weekly; thus 74 treatments were offered each week in seven group sessions.

With regard to time, in 1962–64 therapists' time expended on those who were collected as inpatients, continuing as outpatients, was estimated to be 11 hours/patient, and the mean attendance per patient was 30 group sessions. In 1973, treating mainly those collected as out-patients, the therapists' time per patient was estimated to be 5½ hours and the mean attendance was 17 group sessions per patient.

With regard to the availability of therapists, our otherwise good junior doctors, being Asian, are unsuitable group therapists on grounds of language barriers and cultural differences. One general practitioner, British born and trained in the method as a registrar in psychiatry, takes one group session weekly; one general practitioner, of Middle Eastern origin, with excellent command of the language and under-standing of the culture has recently completed training; he, too, takes a weekly group session. Nursing administration has been unable to provide regular nursing time for training in or practising the method. Three voluntary lay group therapists have been trained in the method. They were originally patients, and during treatment showed a talent for treating their fellows; they were recruited as therapists after completing their treatment. At their wish a doctor sits in at their sessions occasionally and they refer any problems to me.

Group sessions are from 7 to 9 pm, preceded by a relaxation class taken by nursing staff. This appears to be the optimum time in the interests of keeping patients and their spouses at work and obtaining the services of lay therapists.

In April 1976 74 psychotherapeutic treatments were offered each week for the expenditure of two consultant sessions, one clin-ical assistant session and travelling expenses for three lay therap-ists.

It might be expected that this 'conveyor belt' method would carry a high dropout rate. In 1962, collecting inpatients for the Controlled series, the dropout rate was 8 per cent. Patients of both sexes collected mainly as outpatients in 1973 showed a dropout rate amongst neurotics of 12 per cent. In both these years good social worker support was available; without this it is impossible to ascertain the dropout rate, because patients will often discontinue attendance without notice and do so for various reasons, many because they think they are recovered but are not yet confident enough to cross the Rubicon of discharge; in some cases attendance is prevented by practical problems which a social worker might solve, while others should be classified as dropouts. It is perhaps relevant to quote Brill's (1964) dropout rate of 43.5 per cent for both analytical psychotherapy and brief psychotherapy of conventional type.

Conclusion

A course of psychotherapy is beneficial to neurotic patients and, if conducted by this method, is so economical of doctors' time as to render it practicable to offer treatment to all neurotics referred to peripheral hospitals who are suitable as regards age, intelligence and general health. The dropout rate suggests that patients tolerate the method well.

Acknowledgements

The author has pleasure in thanking Dr R. H. Hobson for his help and advice; Dr Paul Rogers and Mr John Lawe for their help in collecting data; those patients, relatives and family doctors without whose co-operation a sufficient number of the series could not have been traced; and Dr R. C. B. Pettigrew for his encouragement.

References

Bovill, D. (1965). *Continuity of Psychotherapy in the Neuroses.* M.D. thesis, London.
Bovill, D. (1972). A trial of group psychotherapy for neurotics. *British Journal of Psychiatry,* **120**, 285–92.
Bovill, D. (1973). Teaching neurotic patients to treat themselves. *Practitioner,* **210**, 679–84.
Brill, N. G. (1964). A comparative study of the effectiveness of psychotherapy. 6th International Congress of Psychotherapy, London.
Sloane, R. B., Staples, F. R., Cristol, A. H., Yorkston, N. J. and Whipple, K. (1975). *Psychotherapy versus Behaviour Therapy.* Cambridge, Mass., and London: Harvard University Press.
Wallace, H. E. R. and Whyte, M. B. H. (1959). The natural history of the psychoneuroses. *British Medical Journal,* i, 144–7.

Diana Bovill, M.D., M.R.C.Psych., *Consultant Psychiatrist, Burnley General Hospital, Casterton Avenue, Burnley, Lancs BB10 2 PQ*

(*Received 8 June 1976; revised 7 January 1977*)

Acknowledgements

My grateful thanks are due to many members of staff of St Crispin Hospital, Northampton during 1961–65, where I started to practise the method and collected the data for the controlled study, especially to Drs Andrew Graham and Paul Rogers, Mr J. Lawe and Mr R. Billingham. To many friends and helpers in Burnley General Hospital and its district during 1973–81, especially to my co-therapists Drs Richard Pettigrew and Ali Syed, Mr J. Keningham, Mr J. Wood, Mrs L. Miller and others. To Mrs L. Miller for typing the manuscript in her spare time and refusing payment. To those who have taken an active part in the management of patients receiving tutorial therapy and in the collection of data for this book, notably Mrs P. Farmer, Mr E. Jaggers, Mrs D. Davenport, Mrs G. Walters and Mrs C. Robinson. To Dr R. H. Hobson for his encouragement with regard to the method and his help in preparation of the book.

References

Adler, A. (1929). *The Practice and Theory of Individual Psychology*. London: Kegan Paul, Trench and Trubner

Atkin, I. (1959). *Br. Med. J.* ii, 1477

Bovill, D. (1965). *Continuity of Psychotherapy in the Neuroses*. MD thesis, London

Bovill, D. (1972). A trial of group psychotherapy for neurotics. *Br. J. Psychiat.*, **120**, 285

Bovill, D. (1977). An outcome study of group psychotherapy. *Br. J. Psychiat.*, **131**, 95

Bovill, D. (1973). Teaching neurotic patients to treat themselves. *The Practitioner*, **210**, 679

Bromberg, W. (1961). *Current Psychiatric Therapies by Masserman Vol 1*, New York and London: Grune and Stratton, pp. 152–8

Dejerine, J. and Gaukler, E. (1911). *Psychoneurosis and Psychotherapy*. Philadelphia and London: Lippincote Co.

Dubois, M. (1913). Le rôle de l'emotion dans la genèse de psychopaties. *Rev. Med. Suissa Romande*, **XXXIII**, 8

Eysenck, H. J. (1960). *Handbook of Abnormal Psychology*. London: Pitman Medical Publishing Co.

Freud, S. (1933). *New Introductory Lectures on Psychoanalysis*. London: Hogarth Press

Hobson, R. H. (1974). Loneliness. *J. Analyt. Psychol.*, **19**, I, 71

Johnson, J. A. (1963). *Group Psychotherapy*. New York: McGraw-Hill Book Co.

Jung, C. G. (1954). *Collected Works*. London: Routledge and Kegan Paul

Lewis, A. (1956). *Price's Text Book of the Practice of Medicine*. Oxford: Oxford University Press

Liddell, H. S. (1954). Conditioning and emotions. *Sci. Amer.*, **190**, 1, 48

Marks, I. (1981). *Br. J. Psychiat.*, **139**, 74

Martin, I. C. *Relaxation*. P.O. Box 99, Chelmsford: Graves Medical Audio-visual Library

Pavlov, I. P. (1926). *Conditioned Reflexes*. London: Constable and Co.

Pratt, J. H. (1945). *Group Psychotherapy by J. L. Moreno*. New York: Beacon House

Rogers, C. R. (1942). *Counselling and Psychotherapy*. New York: Houghton Mifflin

Schilder, F. (1936). *Amer. J. Psychiat.*, **93**, 601

Slavson, S. R. (1947). *The Practice of Group Psychotherapy*. London: Pushkin Press

Wallace, H. E. R. and Whyte, M. B. H. (1959). *Br. Med. J.*, i, 144

Wolf, A. and Swartz, E. K. (1962). *Psychoanalysis in Groups*. New York: Grune and Stratton

Wolpe, J. (1958). *Psychotherapy by Reciprocal Inhibition*. Stanford University Press.

Glossary

This glossary is intended for the convenience of lay readers. Those who are well informed in the subject under discussion are asked to forgive minor inaccuracies, these being due to the need for simplicity and brevity. The meanings given are those relevant to the use of the word in this book.

Abreaction	The emotional reaction resulting from the recall of the original psychic trauma.
Abstem and Antabuse	Medicaments which cause vomiting if alcohol is also taken.
Agoraphobia	Dread of open spaces, in fact usually dread of the people in the open spaces.
Analysis	Psychoanalysis.
Anorexia	Loss of appetite for food.
Anorexia nervosa	Hysterical aversion for food.
Anxiety neurosis	A neurosis characterized by anxious apprehensions.
Behaviourism	School of psychology based on the theory that all behaviour, including abnormal behaviour, is learned, i.e. results from conditioned reflexes. Many now think this an oversimplification.
Behaviour therapy	Treatment, derived from behaviourist theory, directed towards desensitizing, i.e. abolishing conditioned reflexes which are causing distress and/or disability (for description see Kenning-

ham, Chapter 10), often practised by psychologists. Has been described as best suited to neurotic disabilities of a very circumscribed nature.

Brain damage   Damage to the brain which affects emotions or capacity for thinking. Usually due to age, accident, disease or misuse of alcohol.

Chorea   St Vitus Dance. Disease characterized by involuntary and irregular movements.

Claustrophobia   Dread of enclosed spaces, in fact usually dread of the people in the spaces.

Clinical assistant   A physician, commonly one taking sessions in one specialty who is usually employed in another specialty; often a general practitioner taking one or two hospital sessions/week in a specialty in which he has special interest and knowledge.

Closed group   Group psychotherapy for which a fixed number of patients is assembled to start treatment on a given date, and no new patients then join the group. Uneconomical in therapists' time if a number dropout leaving few to attend.

Compulsive eater   One who eats to gain comfort and allay anxiety, and leads to overweight. May alternate, in the same patient, with anorexia nervosa.

Community nurse   One attending discharged hospital patients in their homes.

Conditioned reflex   A reflex is a reaction which occurs for self-preservation automatically and instantaneously, i.e. snatching one's hand back on touching a hotplate. A reflex which has been learned is called a conditioned reflex; for example, when an experienced car driver sees a blockage in the road in front of him he automatically and instantaneously transfers his foot from the accelerator to the brake.

From an early age normal behaviour includes many conditioned reflexes. Pavlov (1926) coined this term and demonstrated that, having established conditioned reflexes in dogs, he could apply them to cause neurotic reactions in dogs. The author and many others believe that conditioned reflexes learned in childhood play an important part in neurosis; for example, an adult's excessive and needless fear of criticism was learned in childhood when criticism inferred parental rejection and led to punishment.

Control
Controlled study

A research term.

If, for example, you wished to test a new kind of washing powder you might wash some whites in it and then wash some similar whites in the old powder in order to compare them. This would be a controlled study on the new powder, the whites washed in the old powder being the controls. No study on a new treatment is fully acceptable without controls.

Cover

The covering of symptoms by the patient so that the doctor does not know about them.

Dementia

Insanity characterized by mental impairment and deterioration.

Depression

A state of lowered mental and physical activity. There are two kinds of depression: (a) Endogenous depression, an affective psychosis, may occur in the same patient alternately with mania or hypomania which are states of heightened mental and physical activity. All are thought to be caused by biochemical changes in the body which are not yet fully understood. (b) Exogenous and/or neurotic depression are caused by circumstances calculated to cause unhappiness, such as bereavement, and/or by the state of neurotic disablement with its attendant social stigma etc. Endogenous depression responds to medicinal and physical treatment but not to psychotherapy. Neurotic depression responds poorly, if at all, to such methods but responds to successful treatment of neurosis by psychotherapy. Different symptoms characterize the two conditions, though they can sometimes be difficult to differentiate. The affective psychoses can occur in the presence of neurosis just as any physical illness can occur in the presence of neurosis.

Desensitize
To abolish conditioned reflexes which are causing distress and/or disability. Practised in behaviour therapy, a description appears under Kenningham, Chapter 10. In tutorial therapy patients are taught to desensitize themselves assisted by an understanding of the original source of the conditioned reflex. Success and failure occur in both methods, and they have not been compared in a controlled study.

Dropouts
Patients who reject a treatment, discontinuing it before it is completed.

Dry
Describes an alcoholic who is no longer taking alcohol.

Follow-up
Review and assessment of patients included in a research study at a stated period after completion of treatment.

Freudian forgetting
Forgetting information and episodes that are unpleasant to remember.

Grade 6
The grade of nurse from which ward sisters and charge nurses are drawn.

Hard drugs
The more dangerous drugs of addiction, for example heroin.

Housebound
Agoraphobia to such a degree that the patient will not leave the house; may be partial or phasic.

Hypertension
High blood pressure.

Hypochondriasis
Morbid anxiety about health. The fear causes exaggeration of minor symptoms, and the patient often becomes convinced that he has a physical disease which his doctors have failed to identify.

Hypomania
See depression.

Hysteria
Usually applied to those who unconsciously seek attention exceptionally, often through hypochondriasis, who are histrionic and who overreact – or underreact – emotionally. They

obtain 'secondary gain', usually in the form of attention.

Hysterical conversion The development of a symptom without physical cause, for example, a paralysis or blindness for which there is no physical cause.

Hysterical reaction Emotionally disordered behaviour or dissociation.

Intelligence quotient (IQ) Intelligence is measured by intelligence tests, and the result is given as a figure which is the quotient. Average adult intelligence is IQ 100, and the bottom limit of adult normal intelligence is usually regarded as IQ 70.

Mania *See* Depression.

Moral deficient An old-fashioned descriptive term for psychopath.

Neurosis A group of mental illnesses which do not amount to, nor lead to, insanity.

Neuroticism Patterns of thinking are reacting which are flaws in the adjustment to life. If a stress related to such a flaw is applied by circumstances neurosis occurs unless the subject's compensations and/or escape mechanisms prove sufficient to 'paper over' the flaw.

Obsessional neurosis Characterized by compulsions leading to rituals; for example, the subject may be unable to wash and dry his hands once but may feel compelled to do so three or nine times, etc.

Open group A group meeting for psychotherapy which has a shifting population. When one patient is discharged another joins. *See* Closed group.

Pathology The cause and effects of diseases so far as they are known.

Personality disorder This term has no precise meaning but is commonly used as a euphemism for the term psychopath.

Phobia Any persistent morbid dread or fear.

Psychiatrist A physician who practises psychiatry.

Psychiatry The branch of medicine which deals with mental and emotional disorders.

Psychic   Pertaining to the mind (*not* pertaining to the supernatural).

Psychoanalysis   A method of psychotherapy. Freud (1933) coined the term which is sometimes used to mean only the Freudian method, but often used to include the methods of Freud's colleagues, Jung (1954) and Adler (1929), who broke away from Freud's school and founded their own schools.

Freud taught that most mental and emotional abnormalities are caused by errors in the sexual development from the moment of birth. He saw infantile suckling and defaecation as being primarily sexual, and sex as being the central theme of human life from the cradle to the grave. In developing a terminology for his theories he borrowed freely from Greek mythology. Adler, however, rejected Freud's sexual theory and taught that neurosis is caused by inferiority feelings implanted in infancy and early childhood, that the pursuit of compensation for these feelings, through success, continues throughout life and neurosis occurs as a result of failure.

Psychologist   One holding a degree in the science of psychology, but who is not usually also qualified as a physician. Medical psychologists are valued ancillary workers in psychiatric units, they undertake testing, such as for intelligence, they are trained in research methods and often practise behaviour therapy.

Psychology   The science of the mind, mental operations and behaviour.

Psychopath   This term has been variously defined: one having a 'Persistent disorder or disability of the mind . . . which results in abnormally aggressive or serious irresponsible conduct' (Mental Health Act 1959).

'Abnormal personalities who cause society to suffer (from their abnormalities)' (Schneider).

The disorder is characterized by lessened voluntary control and increased emotional response to stimuli, by deficiencies of feeling and of ethical sense. Psychopaths differ from the average person only in degree and there are degrees of psychopathy; thus there is no established or recognized borderline between irresponsible conduct and 'seriously irresponsible conduct', it is a matter of degree. The author has defined a psychopath as one having congenitally below-average goodwill.

Psychotherapy   Dejerine (Dejerine and Gaukler, 1911) defined it as 'the influence for good of one mind upon another', which is a comprehensive definition; it includes the work of schoolteachers, ministers of religion, physicians and many others who usually treat neuroticism rather than neurosis, thus performing a valuable service. The definition also stands for psychotherapy practised in psychiatric units for the treatment of those disabled by neurosis. There are many methods all of which overlap at least to some degree, for example, psychoanalysis, client-centred behaviour therapy. Colloquially, psychotherapy is often called 'talking treatment'. The behaviour of the psychotherapist ranges from that of the Freudian psychoanalyst who may remain completely silent throughout a session with a patient or a group (see patient 1, Chapter 9) and, when speaking, confines himself to interpretation, according to Freudian theory, of something which the patient has said, to, at the other end of the scale, the lecture method of Pratt (1945).

Psychotropic medication   Medicaments used in treating the psyche such as sedatives, tranquillisers and antidepressants.

Referral   A patient referred by another physician to the consultant concerned.

Rituals   See obsessional neurosis.

Scapegoat   Originally a goat which was driven out of the community when the Jewish priest had laid the sins of the people upon it. A person bearing blame due to others.

Schizophrenia   A psychosis.

Siblings   Brothers and sisters.

Subnormal mentally   An adult having an intelligence quotient below 70.

Transference   The unconscious transfer to the psycho-therapist, by the patient, of the characteristics and/or attitudes of parents or others important in childhood memories. If his father was a bully the patient may assume bullying in the psycho-therapist where none exists.

Trigger factor   The precipitating factor of a neurotic illness.

The following sources of information were used for this glossary:

Eliot Slater and Martin Roth, *Clinical Psychiatry*
Desmond Curran and Maurice Partridge, *Psychological Medicine*
American Pocket Medical Dictionary, edited by W. A. Newman Dorland
Pears Encyclopedia, edited by M. Barker and C. Cook
The Concise Oxford English Dictionary, edited by H. W. Fowler and F. G. Fowler

Index

abreaction
  definition, 207
  see also self-abreaction
abstem, 152, 207
Adler, A., 9, 154, 181
adolescence
  improvement in self-concept, 23
  rebellious phase, 14
affection, failure to demonstrate, 45
affective psychosis, 151, 153, 209, 210
age range of patients, 148, 150, 163-4
aggression
  avoidance of, *see* inadequacy
  importance of, 38
  of female in defence of young, 30-1
  reaction of over-protected child to, 101
agoraphobia, 125
  behaviour, 77-8
  definition, 207
  definition of 'housebound', 210
  management, 78-80
  symptoms, 25
  see also desensitization
Alcoholics Anonymous, 145, 152
alcoholism, 27, 28
  high mean attendance rate for treatment, 165
  pattern of treatment, 152
  problems of breaking reliance, 39

treatment before tutorial therapy, 69
  treating by use of tutorial therapy, 145
anorexia, definition, 207
anorexia nervosa, 153, 174, 175
  definition, 207
Antabuse, 152, 207
anxiety neurosis, 24-5, 120-4, 124-5
  case history, 113-18
  definition, 207
  with obsessional features, 118-20
assertiveness, 82-3
  appropriate use of, 37
  avoidance of, irritating others, 101
  finding appropriate level, 104
  problems of 'only' child, 99
  rebellion against bullying, 41
attendance at sessions by patients, 33
  problems preventing, 127, 143, 147, 173, 174
authority, attitudes to, 37, 43, 82-3

behaviour therapy, 142, 183
  definition, 207-8
behaviourism, 9
  definition, 207
brain
  damage, definition of, 208
  human related to other mammals 52-3

dreams, 83
during treatment, 136-7
in hysteria, 27
interpretation, 43-4
dropouts from course, 147, 149,
166-7, 195, 203
definition, 210
with additional complications,
171
drug abuse, 26-7, 28, 69, 152
drug dependency, 28-9

eccentricities, harmless, 56
electroconvulsive therapy (ECT),
70
received by controls in trial,
187-8
emotional insecurity
and possessiveness, 55
contributory factors, 22-3
trigger factors, 23-4
emotional support, 107-8
acceptance as mirage, 37
escape mechanisms, 26, 133
learning to abandon, 38
see also, alcoholism
experience, and conditioned
reflexes, 13

failure
acceptance as part of life, 97
against unnecessary standards,
117
as a conditioned reflex, 16
and avoiding loss of nerve, 79
gradual erosion of self-
confidence, 39
neurotic reactions to, 15
overwork due to fear of, 67
see also scapegoats
family history, 64
see also parents
fantasies, in hysteria, 27
fathers, dominance in human
families, 31
see also parents
fear
accepting normal levels of, 91

and loss of concentration, 59-60
built-in limitations, 76
finding socially acceptable way
out, 75, 79
integral part of survival mechanism, 25-6, 74-5
manifestations in hysteria, 127
neurotic, 24-6
of disease, see hypochondriasis
patients' shame of, 75-6
physiological symptoms, 39, 51,
74-5, 76-7
steps in treatment, 74-6
see also, desensitization
females
aggression in defence of young,
30-1
dominated by male in family, 31
unable to fight physically, 31-2
freedom of action, 57
Freud, Sigmund, 18, 212
frigidity, 125

goodwill
above-average in neurotics,
19-20
advantage taken by others, 89
rendering patient vulnerable, 22,
37
group psychotherapy, see Tutorial
Therapy

happiness
learning to cultivate habit, 38
positive attitude to one's assets,
58
health, impairment, 163, 164
history of patient, 62-9
hypochondriasis, 141
definition, 210
factors encouraging, 64
management, 83-6
hysterectomy, depression following, 120, 123
hysteria, 27, 127-9
as escape mechanism, 26
attention-seeking, 19
common behaviour pattern, 129